A Guide to General Dental Practice

Edited by

Nick Priest

Hardev Seehra

and

Murray Wallace

Foreword by
Hew Mathewson
General Dental Practitioner
President of the General Dental Council

Radcliffe Publishing
Oxford • Seattle

Radcliffe Publishing Ltd
18 Marcham Road
Abingdon
Oxon OX14 1AA
United Kingdom

www.radcliffe-oxford.com
Electronic catalogue and worldwide online ordering facility.

British Library Cataloguing in Publication Data

A catalogue record for this book is available from the British Library.

ISBN-10 1 84619 087 8
ISBN-13 978 1 84619 087 2

Typeset by Anne Joshua & Associates, Oxford
Printed and bound by TJ International Ltd, Padstow, Cornwall

Contents

Foreword

The move into general practice is an exciting and challenging step and this guide is one of those things you will never know you needed until you cannot find it. Do keep it safe; it is an incredibly useful collection of information produced by a small group of your colleagues and which thousands of practitioners like you have appreciated time and again. Until such time as you really need it, why not look through it? You will find it helpful and reassuring.

General practice can be the most rewarding of careers, and the more you put into it the more you will enjoy it.

Hew Mathewson
General Dental Practitioner and President of the
General Dental Council
May 2006

Preface

The intention of this *Guide to General Dental Practice* is to assist your start to an enjoyable and fulfilling general dental practice career within the United Kingdom. Primary dental care is a dynamic field and continues to change at a swift pace.

There will be areas within this book which may not have kept pace with all the many rapid changes, particularly the transition from old general dental service contracts to new-style contracts. Users of the book need to be aware that this is intended as a guide and it is recommended to be used in conjunction with other reference books and scientific journals where there may be any doubts about 'current' guidelines. However, I feel that the independent and impartial style of the book, together with a supportive content, will more than compensate.

The *Guide to General Dental Practice* would not exist had it not been for the vision of Richard Gorham. He aimed to produce 'a concise and relevant handbook for . . . practitioners, struggling to make sense of general practice . . .' Sean Gibbs industriously continued the good work of Richard and that of the original ten Wessex-based vocational dental practitioners. Hardev and I are very grateful to the contributors who worked extremely hard to rewrite sections of the book in order to bring it up to date.

I hope that you will keep this book readily available while you are working in general dental practice and use it regularly. Understanding the many areas required for sound patient care and learning the required professional responsibilities will help you to enhance the very important ability to reflect on your professional development.

I wish you every success.

Nick Priest
May 2006

About the editors

Nick Priest is a general dental practitioner, Regional Dental Adviser in Vocational Training, and Dental Adviser for the National Clinical Assessment Service. Having graduated from University College London Dental School in 1981, Nick has over 12 years' experience in vocational training. He set up two dental practices in Cornwall; one was featured as a 'Pride of Practice' in *Dental Practice* magazine. He won the Marsh Midda Prize on completion of Bristol University's Open Learning for Dentists (BUOLD). Nick is studying for a Master's in science in medical education at Bristol University and wishes to encourage newcomers into dental practice to look for new challenges.

Hardev Singh Seehra graduated from King's College London in 2004. He was a vocational dental practitioner between 2004 and 2005 and is currently working in general dental practice in Aldershot. In his spare time, Hardev has been involved in charity work in Vietnam and with Dentaid, offers careers advice in schools, and has designed the website for his dental practice. He aims to broaden his skills with a clinical attachment in hospital. Hardev wishes the very best of luck to new dental graduates and for those joining general dental practice for the first time.

Murray Wallace (Wal) graduated in 1972 at Otago University (New Zealand) and experienced dental practice in New Zealand, Australia and Fiji before settling in England where he owns two practices employing 35 members of staff. His long association with Vocational Training since 1979 sees him employing his fifteenth vocational dental practitioner in 2006. Training of all the team members is an integral part of the practice philosophy as evidenced with 11 staff graduating as hygienists and the practice's first therapist in her final university year. Wal runs nurses' courses in Radiography and Sedation and the practice has six qualified NVQ assessors for in-house training.

A reluctant political life sees him as Chairman of the LDC and the local 'Out of Hours Cooperative' – because 'no one else will do it'!

Regular continuous professional development with a special interest in Sedation and Minor Oral Surgery have led to a mentorship with the Dental Sedation Teachers' Group and membership of the Dental Society for the Advancement of Anaesthesia in Dentistry. Wal offers a very healthy outlook to dentistry by practising a relaxed and balanced approach to professional life.

List of contributors

Louise Bligh
General Dental Practitioner
Southampton

Simon Chaplin-Rogers
General Dental Practitioner
Winchester

Ian Glancey
General Dental Practitioner
Portsmouth

Russel Durham
General Dental Practitioner
Winchester

Bill Flett
General Dental Practitioner
Havant

Huw James
General Dental Practitioner
Blandford

Lucy James
General Dental Practitioner
Dorchester

Raj Rattan
General Dental Practitioner
Oxford

Steven Robinson
Orthodontic Consultant
Portsmouth

Helen Spencer
General Dental Practitioner
Havant

Lynn Stevenson
General Dental Practitioner
Southamptom

Nick Squirrel
General Dental Practitioner
Fleet

Stephen Walker
General Dental Practitioner
Havant

Please note that this book was originally compiled by the Wessex Dental Vocational Practitioners, as listed below:

John Dobson	Jean McGuiness
Claire Hodgson	Andrew Prynne
Alison Kippax	Peter Russell
Eileen Lilley	Peter Saund
Michael Lowdell	Norma Smart

Section 1

1 Law and ethics

The General Dental Council (GDC)

The General Dental Council (GDC) is the regulatory body responsible for the dental profession charged with protecting patients. In June 2005 the council produced new guidance for the dental team. A standard for dental professionals sets out a framework of principles and values within which the dental profession should operate. It provides guidance on how to make decisions within that framework. Six core principles are at the heart of the guidance.

1 Putting patients' interests first and acting to protect them.
2 Respecting patients' dignity and choices.
3 Protecting the confidentiality of patients' information.
4 Co-operating with other members of the dental team and other healthcare colleagues in the interest of the patient.
5 Maintaining your professional knowledge and competence.
6 Being trustworthy.

A dental professional must be prepared to justify their actions, they must be willing and able to demonstrate that they are aware of these principles and have upheld them in their practice of dentistry. Supplementary guidance booklets have been published (*Principles of Patient Consent* and *Principles of Patient Confidentiality*) and further are planned later in 2006 (*Principles of Team Working* and *Principles of Complaint Handling*).

You must read and be familiar with all these, which the GDC will send to you.

The GDC aims to register all dental care professionals and is setting up a private complaints scheme, which was launched on 24 May 2006.

The National Health Service (NHS) complaints scheme is also being looked at closely and a new 'Practice Advice and Support Scheme' (PASS) is being developed. The purpose of this scheme is to help dental practitioners whose performance is causing concern and may result in more serious consequences for that practitioner and their patients unless problems are resolved. The PASS scheme will be initiated by the primary care trust (PCT) clinical governance lead and will be linked with continual professional training by the postgraduate dental deans' involvement. It is hoped it will act as an extra link between practice-based complaints and the disciplinary procedures acting to reduce the cases proceeding to these or GDC involvement. Occasionally, dentists may have increasing patient complaints through ill health, behavioural problems or skill deficits.

The National Clinical Assessment Service (NCAS)

The National Clinical Assessment Service (NCAS), previously the National Clinical Assessment Authority (NCAA), was established as a special health authority in April 2001, following recommendations made in the Chief Medical Officer for England's report, *Support Doctors, Protecting Patients* (November 1999) and *Assuring the Quality of Medical Practice: Implementing Supporting Doctors, Protecting Patients* (January 2001). In April 2003 the NCAS expanded its services to include salaried dentists and from April 2005 has provided a full service to all NHS dentists.

In order to help practitioners in difficulty, NCAS provides advice, takes referrals and carries out targeted assessment where necessary. The NCAS's assessment involves trained medical and lay assessors. Once an objective assessment has been carried out, NCAS will advise on the appropriate course of action. NCAS does not take over the role of an employer, nor does it function as a regulator.

NCAS is established as an advisory body, and the NHS employer organisation remains responsible for resolving the problem once the NCAS has produced its assessment.

The NCAS Advice Service can be accessed 24 hours a day. NCAS is not set up to take referrals directly from the public. This is because performance management needs the active co-operation of the employing authority, as they must take ownership of the situation. www.ncaa.nhs.uk.

Complaints

Many instances of patient dissatisfaction never develop into a complaint because the dentist gives a prompt explanation or a courteous apology.

Since April 1996, every practice providing NHS treatment has had to have an in-house complaints procedure (NHS (GDS) Amendment Regulations 1996). Complaints should be acknowledged in writing within three working days of receipt, and a full response should be made within ten working days of receipt, following a full investigation. If there is to be a delay in the investigation and full response, for example because a member of staff involved in the patient's care is on holiday, the patient should be informed of the reason for the delay, and when to expect a response.

The practice complaints officer or dentist responsible for the patient's treatment should give an explanation, an apology if appropriate and an indication of the action that will be taken to remedy the situation and to make sure that it does not happen again. The GDC endorses the NHS Executive and British Dental Association (BDA) guidance on handling complaints.

The patient is always entitled to a prompt, sympathetic and, above all, accurate account of the facts. An appropriate apology is an act of common courtesy and not admission of liability. Most patients who are given a prompt explanation and apology do not pursue their complaint or make a claim for compensation.

Communication

In the Dental Defence Union's (DDU) experience, complaints and claims seldom arise solely from problems with clinical management. They can be caused by deficiencies in administration systems, procedures and lines of communication. The GDC expects dentists to provide a high standard of care. Failures in communication or organisational systems can have an impact on the delivery of high-quality healthcare. Clear paths of communication are essential between you and:

- your patients
- the dental nurse
- the receptionist
- the laboratory
- all other members of the dental team.

In general, good communication with patients is aided by:

- not talking down to patients – treat them as equals
- allowing patients to state their problems, listening and allowing them to ask questions

- avoiding the use of dental jargon – explain things clearly or draw a diagram and always ask patients if they have understood
- keeping detailed notes of all communications with patients
- treating patients as you would wish to be treated yourself.

Confidentiality

Confidentiality has always been a cornerstone of good dental practice. The GDC's 'Standards Guidance'[1] states:

> The dentist/patient relationship is founded on trust and a dentist should not disclose to a third party information about a patient acquired in a professional capacity without the permission of the patient. To do so may lead to a charge of serious professional misconduct.

The vast majority of cases of breach of confidentiality occur inadvertently, for example where a conversation is overheard in a lift or at a reception desk. It is essential that members of the practice are constantly vigilant.

- The dentist/patient relationship is founded on trust.
- Do not discuss patients or their treatment in places where you might be overheard (e.g. reception area, lift).
- Generally, you should not disclose information about a patient to a third party without the patient's permission, preferably in writing.

There are some exceptions to the rule:

- consent – if a patient requests/agrees you may disclose information
- statutory duty and public interest
- information to relatives or carers – when in the patient's best

interest, but generally the patient's consent should be obtained

- a court order.

However, discuss individual cases with your defence organisation.

Consent

A competent adult patient has a fundamental right to give, or withhold, consent to examination, investigation or treatment. Any treatment or investigation, or even deliberate touching carried out without consent, may amount to battery. This could result in an action for damages, or even criminal proceedings, and in a finding of serious professional misconduct by the GDC.

- You should obtain consent before the proposed procedure.
- A patient sitting voluntarily in a dental chair implies consent to an examination, nothing else. Before taking a radiograph, administering local analgesia etc., this must be explained to the patient and expressed consent obtained.
- Consent must be freely given. It may not be valid if it is obtained under duress.
- The patient should understand the treatment that is proposed, and be made aware of any alternatives. An estimate should be given of the fees.
- Explain any risks that may be associated with the treatment, including any foreseeable complications. Explain the option of no treatment.
- The age of consent in the UK is 16, while the age of majority is 18. In some cases patients aged under 16 can give valid consent to dental treatment (so-called 'Gillick' competence).

- Children under the age of 16 should normally attend with a parent or close relative. If the child understands the nature, purpose and risks of treatment, it may be appropriate to continue. Essential emergency treatment may be performed without authority in the patient's best interest. In such a situation seek dento-legal advice.

Treatment

It is the responsibility of the dentist to explain clearly to the patient the nature of the consultation and in particular whether the patient is being accepted for treatment under a particular scheme, including the NHS. The charge for an initial consultation and the probable cost of the subsequent treatment must be made clear to the patient at the outset.

   Checklist:

- Have you checked the medical history?
- Do you know what you are going to do?
- Is it the correct treatment on the correct tooth?
- Does the patient understand and consent to what is to be done?
- Does the patient know how the treatment is to be done?
- If appropriate, has the patient been warned of potential post-operative problems?

Infection control*

The GDC expects appropriate measures to ensure patient safety, which include infection control.

* Refer to BDA advice sheet A12.

The DDU advises dentists to ensure their practice has an infection-control policy tailored to the practice's routines and updated regularly. Implementing safe and realistic infection-control procedures requires the full compliance of the whole dental team. These procedures should be monitored regularly during clinical sessions and discussed at practice meetings.

- All blood and body fluids must be regarded as infective material.
- Check working area is properly prepared.
- Lay out the appropriate equipment.
- Put on a face mask and protective glasses.
- Hand washing and gloving.
- Don't open drawers or touch surfaces or other equipment that have been sterilised/disinfected once contact with patient is established.
- Dispose of needles and sharps and contaminated clinical waste in specified receptacles.

Records

Patients' records are perhaps the most basic of clinical tools, involved in virtually every consultation. They are meant to give a clear and accurate picture of the patient's care and treatment and to help in that treatment. Dental records:

- must be legible, up to date and contemporaneous
- should include an accurate and up-to-date medical history
- should never be erased, overwritten or inked out – errors should be scored out with a single line and corrections should be dated and initialled

- should be available for patients to see – they have rights to access under the Data Protection Act 1998
- should ensure radiographs are of good diagnostic value, accurately labelled and mounted properly.

It is essential to check and record the patient's medical history (negative responses as well as positive responses should be recorded) and to keep detailed notes of any treatments. If you have a computerised records system, make sure you record exactly the same information that you keep in paper records. The NHS FP25 record card is much smaller than the majority of hospital records, but your notes should still be clear and concise. In some circumstances listed in the NHS Statement of Dental Remuneration, NHS patients will also need an NHS treatment plan form (FP17DC) to indicate the cost of their treatment. Failure to provide this may be a breach of terms of service.

Be aware

It is now your responsibility to professionally, legally and ethically analyse, justify and reflect on your actions.

Complaints, discipline, appeals

See Figure 1.1.

Notes

1   All but trivial convictions involving dentists are reported to the GDC by the police and courts.

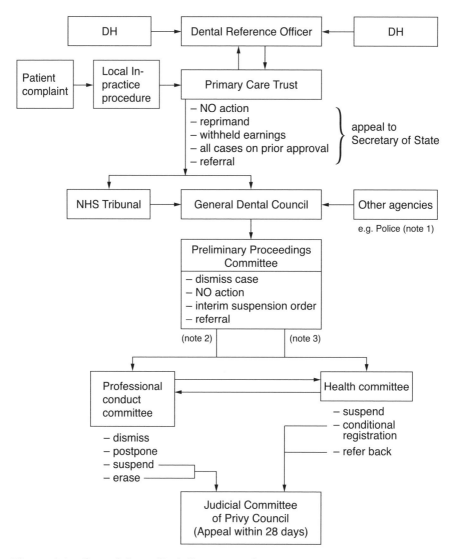

Figure 1.1   Complaints, discipline, appeals.

2   The Professional Conduct Committee deals with all other cases. It meets in March and September each year. Its most serious decision can be erasure from the dental register.

3   The Health Committee was set up by the Dentists' Act of 1984 for cases where fitness or ability to practise is impaired

by physical or mental state. The Committee may then limit registration of a dentist under certain conditions for up to three years, or suspend him or her for no more than a year.

Sample examples of serious professional misconduct:

- operator/anaesthetist resulting in injury or death
- indecent assault
- fraud
- inadequate sterilisation resulting in illness or death.

For further information refer to GDC publications.

Restoration of name

Following suspension or erasure, application can be made not less than ten months after the verdict or ten months after the last rejected appeal for restoration.

The coroner

England and Wales

- The majority of coroners are practising solicitors – some are both medical practitioners and barristers.
- Inquiries into:
  - violent, suspicious or unexplained deaths, unnatural or sudden death of which the cause is unknown
  - death in prison
  - removal of corpses from the country
  - ownership of treasure trove.

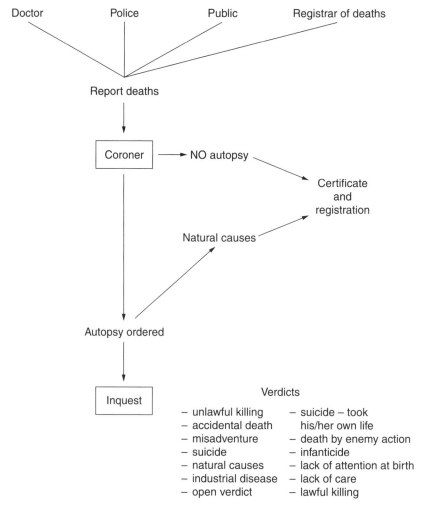

Figure 1.2   Routes of information involved with a coroner's inquiry.

- The coroner may convene an inquest, and must do so in certain circumstances.
- The coroner may summon medical, dental and other witnesses.
- The coroner should be informed:
  - when no doctor has treated the deceased for his/her last illness

- when the doctor attending did not see the deceased within 14 days preceding death or following death
- when death occurred during an operation or before recovery (or within 24 hours) where any form of treatment, including drug therapy, minor operations under local anaesthetic (LA) and dental procedures may be suspected of having some relevance to having contributed to or accelerated death
- when the death was sudden and unexplained or attended by suspicious circumstances
- when the death might be due to an industrial injury, disease or accident, violence, neglect, abortion or to any kind of poisoning.

See Figure 1.2 for a flow diagram showing routes of information involved with a coroner's inquiry.

Reference

1 General Dental Council (2005) General Dental Practice Standards Guidance. GDC, London. www.gdc-uk.org

2 Clinical governance

Raj Rattan

Introduction

In England and Wales, clinical governance (CG) is the vehicle for the delivery of quality healthcare in the NHS. The Labour government introduced the concept in 1997 in the white paper *The New NHS: modern, dependable.*[1] It came about as a result of various NHS scandals through the 1990s, but concerns were expressed about the purpose and process.

David Haslam, a general practitioner (GP) and respected writer from Cambridgeshire, noted that:

> The concept of clinical governance has become something as unwelcome as a dental check-up. We know that we have to do it, we know that it is really for the best, but we simply cannot dig deep and find any enthusiasm for the process.

Neville Goodman, a consultant anaesthetist in Bristol, wrote that:

> the most important elements in the delivery of quality in healthcare are contained in the relations between human beings. With good working relationships clinical governance happens naturally; with poor working relations, setting up committees and defining quality on bits of paper delivers only bits of paper.[2]

A duty of quality was placed on NHS organisations in the 1999 NHS Act. In Section 18(1) it states that 'It is the duty of each Health Authority, Primary Care Trust and NHS trust to put and keep in place arrangements for the purpose of monitoring and improving the quality of health care which it provides to individuals.'

This Act introduced corporate accountability for clinical quality and performance. Clinical governance is described as a 'whole system' process with the following features.

- Patient-centred care needs are at the heart of every NHS organisation. This means that patients are kept well informed and are given the opportunity to participate in their care.
- Good information about the quality of services is available to those providing the services as well as to patients and the public.
- Variations in the process, outcomes and in access to health-care are greatly reduced.
- NHS organisations and partners work together to provide quality-assured services and drive forward continuous improvement.
- Health professionals work in teams to a consistently high standard and identify ways to provide safer and even better care for their patients.
- Risks and hazards to patients are reduced to as low a level as possible, creating a safety culture throughout the NHS.
- Good practice and research evidence is systematically adopted.

It was as a result of this that, in 2001, it became a requirement for dentists practising in the NHS to have a quality-assurance system in place. The new dental contract in 2006 places further emphasis on this requirement.

More recently, the Health and Social Care (Community Health and Standards) Act 2003 refers to the 'duty of quality' and states that it is the duty of each NHS body to put and keep in place arrangements for the purpose of monitoring and improving the quality of healthcare provided by and for that body.

Definition

Clinical governance is a system through which NHS organisations are accountable for continuously improving the quality of their services and safeguarding high standards of care by creating an environment in which excellence in clinical care will flourish (*see* Figure 2.1).

Roy Lilley, a prolific writer on healthcare matters, took the view that it was about 'doing anything and everything required to maximise quality'.[3]

The Royal College of General Practitioners defines it in relation to activities by describing it as 'a framework for the improvement of patient care through commitment to high standards, reflective practice, risk management, and personal and team development'.[4]

The underlying principles of CG were first set out in *The New NHS: modern, dependable*.[1] These are:

1 evidence-based practice
2 the dissemination of good ideas in practice
3 quality-improvement processes
4 use of high-quality data to monitor clinical care
5 clinical risk-reduction programmes
6 investigation of adverse events
7 learning from complaints
8 dealing with poor performance
9 implementation of professional development programmes
10 leadership skill development.

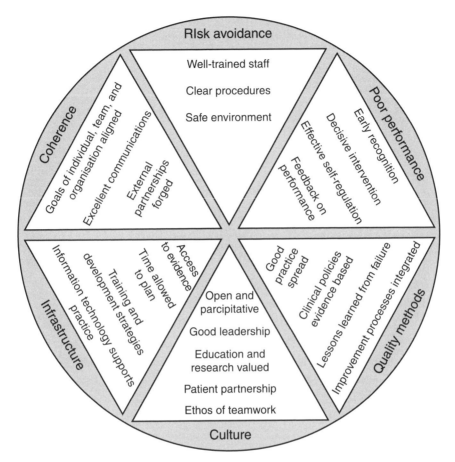

Figure 2.1 Approaches to clinical governance. *Source*: Scally G and Donaldson L (1998) Looking forward: clinical governance and the drive for quality improvement in the new NHS in England. *BMJ*. **317** (7150): 61–5.

In this publication, the Department of Health has clearly stated the importance of quality control in the NHS by stating that:

> every part of the NHS and everyone who works in it should take responsibility for working to improve quality. This must be quality in the broadest sense; doing the right thing at the right time for the right people and doing them right – first time. And it must be quality of the patient's experience as well as the clinical result – quality measured

in terms of prompt access, good relationships and efficient administration.

Aims

CG sets out to ensure that:

- systems to monitor the quality of clinical practice are in place and are functioning properly
- clinical practice is reviewed and improved as a result
- practitioners meet standards, such as those issued by the national professional regulatory bodies
- practitioners adhere to best-practice guidelines

The idea is to raise standards generally which means pushing the profession's whole performance profile up. As dentists recognise something as good practice, and define it as a guideline, so more dentists will adopt the practice, thereby shifting the mean standards of practice (*see* Figure 2.2).

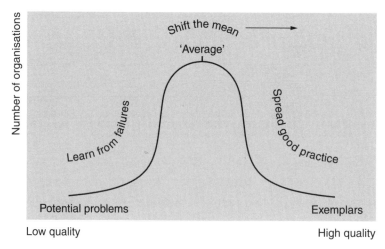

Figure 2.2   The spread of good practice.

Government agencies

As part of its drive for quality in healthcare, the British government has created a number of organisations.

National Patient Safety Agency (NPSA)

The NPSA is a special health authority created in July 2001 to co-ordinate the efforts of the entire country to report, and more importantly to learn from, mistakes and problems that affect patient safety. It encourages all healthcare staff to report incidents without undue fear of personal reprimand and has recently launched its publication *Medical Error* to redouble its efforts in this respect.

Examples of its advisory work relevant to dentistry include the information published in May 2005 on how to better protect patients with latex allergy. This is available from the NPSA website.

NICE

The National Institute for Health and Clinical Excellence (NICE) is a special health authority for England and Wales. Its role is to provide patients and health professionals with 'authoritative, robust and reliable guidance on current "best practice"'. NICE guidance covers three areas.

1   Clinical guidelines cover the appropriate treatment and care of patients with specific diseases and conditions within the NHS in England and Wales.
2   Technology appraisals cover the use of new treatments within the NHS in England and Wales.

3   Interventional procedures cover the safety and efficacy of interventional procedures for diagnosis and treatment.

The publications relevant to dentistry are

- *Guidance on Removal of Third Molars*[5]
- *Guidance on Recall Intervals*[6]
- *Use of HealOzone in the Treatment of Pit and Fissure Caries and Root Caries.*[7]

The Healthcare Commission

The Healthcare Commission (HC) is the name of the independent inspectorate body for the NHS in England; the legal name is the 'Commission for Healthcare Audit and Inspection'.

It was formed by the Health and Social Care (Community Health and Standards) Act 2003, and launched on 1 April 2004. It replaces and takes over the functions of a number of regulators of the NHS including its predecessor, the Commission for Health Improvement (CHI). Its range of responsibilities is aimed at improving the quality of healthcare. It has a statutory duty to:

- assess the management, provision and quality of NHS healthcare and public health services
- review the performance of each NHS trust
- regulate the independent healthcare sector through registration, annual inspection, monitoring complaints and enforcement
- publish information about the state of healthcare
- consider complaints about NHS organisations that the organisations themselves have not resolved

- promote the co-ordination of reviews and assessments carried out by ourselves and others
- carry out investigations of serious failures in the provision of healthcare.

In carrying out its duties, the Commission is required to pay particular attention to:

- the availability of, access to, quality and effectiveness of healthcare
- the economy and efficiency of the provision of healthcare
- the availability and quality of information provided to the public about healthcare
- the need to safeguard and promote the rights and welfare of children and the effectiveness of measures taken to do so.

It should be emphasised that the powers of the Commission extend beyond the NHS and include the independent (non-NHS) sector. It will regulate independent dentists who provide listed services, as described in the Private and Voluntary Healthcare Regulations (England) 2001. Listed services include class 3b (except where such treatment is carried out by, or under of the supervision of, a healthcare professional), class 4 lasers and intense pulsed light sources. The Commission urges:

> unregistered dentists who currently provide these services to make application for registration to the Healthcare Commission without delay. It is an offence under section 11(i) of the Care Standards Act 2000 to carry on or manage an establishment that provides registerable services without being registered. Continuing to provide such services may lead to prosecution.[8]

The seven-domain framework

As of April 2005, the approach of the Healthcare Commission to quality assurance and standards setting has been to create a framework that is common to all of healthcare and includes general dental practice – one framework to be populated with criteria and guidance specific to each branch of healthcare. Driven by the publication *Standards for Better Health*,[8] which sets out the level of quality all organisations providing NHS care will be expected to meet or aspire to across the NHS in England, it puts quality firmly at the forefront of the agenda for the NHS.

The focus is on providing a common set of requirements, expressed as core and development standards, applying across all healthcare organisations to ensure that health services are provided that are both safe and of an acceptable quality; there is also emphasis on the process of continuous quality improvement.

The 23 core standards describe the level of quality that healthcare organisations, including dental practices, will be expected to meet. The standards are organised into seven domains.

Safety

How do we manage and minimise risk in the practice? What systems and processes do we have in place to ensure patient safety?

Clinical and cost effectiveness

How are we ensuring that patients receive care and treatment that meet their individual needs? Do we apply research evidence to provide effective clinical outcomes?

Governance

How are we dealing with managerial responsibility, clinical leadership and professional accountability? What is the culture within the practice? What systems and working practices do we have in place to ensure that probity, quality assurance, quality improvement and patient safety are among the pillars of our practising philosophy?

Patient focus

How can we show that the services we provide are patient-centred? Are we respecting their diverse needs, preferences and choices? Are we working collaboratively with other organisations, like the secondary care sector or the community dental services to ensure the patient journey is seamless?

Accessible and responsive care

Are patients receiving services as promptly as possible? Do they have a choice in access to services and treatments they receive? Do they experience unnecessary delays at any stage of service delivery?

Care environment and amenities

What is the physical environment like where patients are treated? Is it conducive to the well-being of patients and staff? Does it show respect for patients' needs and preferences?

Is there adequate privacy? Are treatment rooms and waiting rooms well maintained, hygienic and clean?

Public health

How can we show that programmes and services are designed and delivered in collaboration with all relevant organisations and communities? How do we promote, protect and improve the health of the population at large to reduce health inequalities between different population groups and areas?

The core standards set out the minimum level of service that patients have a right to expect and the developmental standards signal the direction of travel for future planning and delivery to reflect increasing patient expectations. The HC is resolute about the framework, stating that 'meeting the core standards is not optional'.

In addition to the core standards, there are a number of developmental standards which reflect the increasing drive towards continuous quality improvement in the NHS.

The Department of Health has published guidance for dentists on how the Healthcare Commission framework can be applied in the general practice setting. The core standards are grouped under 12 themes all of which relate to general dental practice. These are:

1   Infection control.
2   Child protection.
3   Dental radiography.
4   Staff, patient, and environmental safety.
5   Evidenced-based practice and research.
6   Prevention and public health.
7   Clinical records, patient privacy and confidentiality.
8   Staff involvement and development (for all staff).

9 Clinical staff requirements and development.

10 Patient information and involvement.

11 Fair and accessible care.

12 Clinical audit and peer review.

The reader is referred to http://www.pcc.nhs.uk/142.php where a copy of the framework is available for download.

References

1 Department of Health (1997) *The New NHS: Modern, Dependable*. Department of Health, London.

2 Goodman N (1998) Clinical governance. *BMJ*. **317**: 1725–7.

3 Lilley R (1999) *Making Sense of Clinical Governance*. Radcliffe Medical Press, Oxford.

4 Royal College of General Practitioners (1999) *Practice Advice on the Implementation of Clinical Governance in England and Wales*. RCGP, London.

5 National Institute for Clinical Excellence (2000) *Guidance on Removal of Third Molars*. NICE Technology Appraisal No. 1. **March**. NICE, London.

6 National Institute for Clinical Excellence (2004) *Guidance on Recall Intervals*. NICE Clinical Guide No. 19. **October**. NICE, London.

7 National Institute for Clinical Excellence (2005) *Use of HealOzone in the Treatment of Pit and Fissure Caries and Root Caries*. NICE Technology Appraisal No. 092. **July**. NICE, London.

8 Healthcare Commission. *Standards for Better Health.* www.healthcarecommission.org.uk

Section 2

3 Medical histories

Suggested medical history form

See Table 3.1 for a suggested medical history form.

Assessment of the patient's medical history

Many systems have been devised to ascertain a thorough medical history. The following is given as an example.

1 Anaemia:
   - contraindication to general anaesthetic (GA)
   - breathlessness, lassitude, weakness
   - racial origins – haemolytic anaemia.
2 Bleeding disorders:
   - history of family involvement
   - history of previous difficulty in achieving haemostasis.
3 Cardio-respiratory disorders:
   - contraindication to GA
   - may require antibiotic cover
   - rheumatic fever, ischaemic heart disease, cardiac operations
   - wheeze, cough, dyspnoea
   - aspirin cover.

Table 3.1   Suggested medical history form.

In order to provide you with the most appropriate and safest treatment, your dentist needs to know about any previous or current medical conditions since many of them can affect your dental treatment. Completion of this questionnaire will help us to help you and together we will update your records at each new course of treatment.

ALL DETAILS WILL BE STRICTLY CONFIDENTIAL

Surname: _____

Forname(s): _____ Title: _____

Sex: Male/Female _____

Date of birth: _____ day _____ month _____ year

Address: _____

_____

_____ Postcode: _____

Telephone: (Home) _____ (Work) _____

Referred by: _____

Date of last dental treatment: _____

Occupation: _____

Doctor's name _____

Address: _____

_____

_____

Doctor's telephone number: _____

Table 3.1   (*cont.*)

Questions	Yes	No	Details
DO YOU:			
1. Have allergies to any medicines e.g. antibiotics, substances e.g. latex or foods?			
2. Have hay fever or eczema?			
3. Have arthritis?			
4. Have a heart pacemaker?			
5. Have diabetes, or does anyone in your family?			
6. Suffer fainting attacks, giddiness or blackouts?			
7. Bruise easily or have persistent bleeding following injury, tooth extraction or surgery?			
8. Have any infectious diseases (including HIV or hepatitis)?			
9. Take, or have you taken, steroids?			
ARE YOU CURRENTLY:			
1. Pregnant?			
2. Receiving treatment from a doctor, hospital or clinic?			
3. Taking any prescribed medicines (e.g. tablets, ointments, injections, inhalers including contraceptives or hormone replacement therapy)?			
4. Carrying a warning card?			
DID YOU, as a child, or since have:			
1. Growth hormone treatment before the mid 1980s?			
2. Heart surgery?			
3. Brain surgery?			
4. Rheumatic fever or chorea (St Vitus Dance)?			
5. Liver disease (e.g. jaundice, hepatitis) or kidney disease?			
6. Any other serious illness?			

Table 3.1 (*cont.*)

Questions	Yes	No	Details
DID YOU, as a child, or since have:			
7. Blood refused by the Blood Transfuction Service?			
8. A bad reaction to general or local anaesthetic?			
9. A joint replacement or other implant?			
10. Treatment that required you to be in hospital?			
DRINKING: How many units of alcohol do you drink per week? (A unit of alcohol is approximately half a pint of lager, a single measure of spirits, or a single glass of wine/aperitif).			_____ units per week
SMOKING AND CHEWING:			
Do you smoke any tobacco products now, or in the past?			_____ per day
Do you chew tobacco, betel-quid, gutkha or supari now, or in the past?			_____ per day

Please give any other details, which your dentist might need to know about, such as self-prescribed medicine (e.g. aspirin)

_____

_____

Completed by: (Please tick)   Self: ☐   Parent: ☐   Guardian: ☐

I agree to this information being made available to other healthcare professionals as may be necessary.

Signature: _____ Date: _____

Medical History Update: Please check that the health information on this form is still correct (including information on smoking and drinking), if not, amend as necessary, or note any changes below.

Date	No Change	List Any Changes Below	Patient's Initials

4   Drug treatment and allergy:
- corticosteroids
- antihypertensives
- anticonvulsants
- anticoagulants
- antidiabetics
- antibiotics
- contraceptives (prescribed drugs may cause pill failure)
- drug abuse
- history of any antibiotic resistance
- chemotherapy agents
- immunosuppressants.

5 Endocrine disorders:
- diabetes mellitus
- hyperthyroidism
- hypoadrenocorticism

6 Fits or faints:
- epilepsy
- other causes.

7 Gastro-intestinal disorders:
- Crohn's
- coeliac disease
- vomiting
- abdominal pain.

8 Hospital admissions:
- previous operations
- underlying disease
- Creutzfeldt-Jacob disease.

9 Jaundice and liver disease:
- hepatitis B
- impaired drug metabolism.

10 Kidney disorders:
- drug excretion impairment
- hypertension.

11 Likelihood of pregnancy:
- contraindication to routine radiography
- care in drug prescription.

12 Social history:
- lifestyle
- high-risk infectious disease
- nature of work.

13 Risk of oral cancer:
- smoking
- heavy drinking
- chewing betel nut or tobacco
- immunocompromised
- previous history.

Implications of common medical problems

Central nervous system

Headache and facial pain

- Local causes – dental disease, infections (sinusitis).
- Psychogenic – tension headache, temporomandibular joint (TMJ) dysfunction.
- Vascular – migraine, migrainous neuralgia, temporal arteritis.
- Neurological – trigeminal/glossopharyngeal neuralgia, intracranial lesions.

- Miscellaneous – referred cardiac pain, Paget's disease, raised intracranial pressure.

Cerebrovascular accidents

- Hemiplegia – facial palsy.
- Speech/comprehension difficulty.
- Impaired mobility/manual dexterity.
- Hypertension – anticoagulants.

Epilepsy

- Dental trauma:
  - mucosal scarring
  - lacerations to mouth/tongue.
- Possible contraindication to dentures, complex restorations and some orthodontic therapy.
- Gingival hyperplasia (phenytoin).
- Occasional psychiatric problems.
- Subluxation of TMJ.

Depression

- TMJ dysfunction syndrome.
- Atypical facial pain.
- Oral dysaesthesis (burning mouth, sore tongue).

Down's syndrome

- Delayed eruption – irregular sequence – morphological variation.
- Immune defects – periodontal disease.
- Cardiac defects – infective endocarditis risk.
- Hepatitis B risk.

Cardiovascular system

Heart disease

- Shortness of breath when supine.
- Avoid stress – consider sedation or relative analgesia.
- Hypertension and ischaemic heart disease – possible risk of adrenaline in local anaesthesia, dysrhythmia (minimum dose).
- Angina – ensure patient's glyceryl trinitrate is at hand.
- Possible use of anticoagulants.
- Implanted pacemakers – beware ultrasonic scalers and diathermy.

Infective endocarditis

- Patients at risk:
  - previous episode (high risk)
  - rheumatic valvular disease
  - prosthetic valves
  - congenital cardiac defects (excluding heart murmurs).
- Prophylaxis
  - *one* hour pre-op amoxycillin 3 g, or 600 mg clindamycin one hour pre-op (current prophylactic regimes are under review and readers are advised to refer to the latest *BNF*).

Anaemia

- Atrophic glossitis – sore tongue.
- Predisposition to/exacerbation of candidiasis – angular cheilitis.
- Apthous stomatitis.

Anticoagulant therapy

- Surgical risk – extractions under medical supervision.
- Avoid aspirin and other non-steroid anti-inflammatory drugs (NSAIDs).
- Avoid prolonged broad-spectrum antibiotic therapy.
- Dialysis patients – surgery on the day following dialysis.
- Avoid inferior dental nerve blocks.

Haemophilia

- Surgical risk – extractions planned with medical assessment essential.
- Bleeding risk with intramuscular injections (including inferior dental blocks).
- Avoid aspirin and other NSAIDs.
- Routine dental care – avoid minor trauma.
- Scaling – antihemophilic factor (AHF) cover – preventive advice/procedures important.
- Hepatitis B/AIDS (acquired immune deficiency syndrome) risk.
- Preventive care.

Respiratory system

Chronic

- Chronic obstructed airways disease (COAD) – chronic bronchitis, emphysema.
- Avoid sedation – local anaesthesia only.
- Treat upright.

Asthma

- Reduce anxiety – possible relative analgesia, but no intravenous (IV) sedation.
- Avoid aspirin, paracetamol, mefenamic acid (possible anaphylaxis).
- Awareness of other possible allergies e.g. penicillin.
- Bronchodilators – dry mouth.
- Occasional systemic steroid therapy.

Gastro-intestinal system

Dry mouth

- Causes:
  - anxiety
  - dehydration
  - drugs
  - systemic disease/syndromes
  - radiotherapy.
- Effects:
  - discomfort and denture problems
  - disturbed taste, speech, swallowing
  - tendency to periodontal disease and caries
  - tendency to candidiasis/ascending bacterial sialadenitis.

Oral/denture hygiene

- Palliative drinks/salivary substitutes.
- Fluoride mouth rinses.

Peptic ulceration

- Avoid erosion of teeth due to regurgitation.
- Anaemia.
- Avoid NSAIDs.
- IV sedation – diazepam activity enhanced by cimetidine.

Coeliac disease

- Apthae – glossitis.
- Burning mouth – angular cheilitis.

Crohn's disease

- Mucosal 'tags' or 'cobblestone' proliferation of mucosa.
- Oral ulceration.
- Steroid/immunosuppressive therapy.

Liver

Obstructive jaundice
- Surgical risk of bleeding tendency (due to vitamin K malabsorption).

Cirrhosis
- Surgical risk of bleeding tendency.
- Anaemia.
- Impaired drug metabolism.
- Congenital:
    - green discolouration of teeth
    - hypoplasia.

Hepatitis B or hepatitis C risk

- Known infectious/carrier.
- IV drug abuse.
- Homosexual.
- Geographic risk areas.
- Institutionalised patients.
- Chronic use of blood or blood products.

Management

- Cross-infection control.
- Immunisation.
- Antigen testing.

Kidney

Chronic renal failure

- Impaired drug excretion.
- Hypertension, anaemia, bleeding tendency.
- Anticoagulant therapy following dialysis.
- Immunosuppressed/steroid therapy – transplant patients.
- Candidiasis.
- Some drugs are nephrotoxic e.g. tetracycline.
- Infective risk patients.

Musculo-skeletal

Rheumatoid arthritis

- Painful, swollen joints – possible unstable neck.
- Sjörgren's syndrome.
- Oral drug reactions – lichenoid, oral ulceration.

- Steroid therapy – immunosuppressive candidiasis.
- Anaemia.

Paget's disease

- Enlargement of alveolar ridges.
- Hypercementosis/ankylosis of teeth.
- Difficult and/or traumatic extractions likely with osteomyelitis if appropriate antibiotic therapy is not implemented.
- Occasional pulpal calcification.

Endocrine

Diabetes

- Dry mouth.
- Candidiasis.
- Lichenoid drug reactions.
- Poor response to infection.
- Dental infections may affect control of blood glucose levels.
- Antimicrobials required for oro-facial infections.
- Plan appointments and treatment to minimise risk of hypoglycaemia.

Thyrotoxicosis

- Irritable/anxious patient.
- Tremor, heart failure.
- Possible risk of dysrhythmia with adrenaline LA.
- Dental infections – use antimicrobials and drainage to avoid precipitating crisis.

Hypothyroidism

- Slow reactions/cerebration and poor memory.
- Hypotension, bradycardia.
- Avoid sedation/codeine.

Pregnancy

- Avoid radiography in first and third trimester.
- Avoid drugs.
- Dental treatment if necessary in second trimester.
- 'Pregnancy gingivitis' and epulides.
- Supine hypotension.
- Also check with text before prescribing if mother is breast feeding.
- Avoid removing amalgam fillings.

Oral contraceptives

- Decreased contraceptive effect with certain drug therapy.
- Possible increased tendency to periodontal disease.
- Possible increased risk of dry socket.

Steroid therapy

- Masking of disease processes.
- Opportunistic infections – candidiasis.
- Impaired healing.
- Diabetes.
- Psychosis.
- Osteoporosis.
- Peptic ulceration.

- Cushinoid features.
- Prolonged adrenal atrophy – slow withdrawal of therapy essential.
- Circulatory collapse under stress – dental treatment?

Note: supplementary steroid cover
- IV hydrocortisone sodium succinate 100–200 mg *one* hour pre-op (minor), or
- 20 mg prednisolone (4 mg dexamethasone) *four* hours pre-op + *four* hours post-op.

For more comprehensive information, including general anaesthetic considerations, refer to texts such as:

- Scully C and Cawson RA (1987) *Medical Problems in Dentistry* (2e). Wright, Bristol.

Oral manifestations of drugs

Effects on:

- teeth
- mucosa
- salivary glands.

Teeth

Discolouration

- Extrinsic:
  - smoking
  - iron
  - mouthwashes.

- Intrinsic:
  - tetracyclines
  - fluorides.

Effects on teeth

- Caries – sugars.
- Erosion – acids.
- Abrasion – tooth cleansers.

Mucosa

Keratosis

- Smoking.
- Betel nut chewing
- 'Skaol bandits.'

Burns

- Chemicals.
- Reaction to denture cleansers.
- Aspirin.

Oral candidiasis

- Broad-spectrum antimicrobials.
- Corticosteroids.
- Drugs causing xerostomia.

Herpes virus infection

- Immunosuppressives.

Oral ulceration

- Cytotoxics.
- Gold.
- Penicillamine.
- Phenylbutazone.
- NSAIDs.

Erythema multiforme

- Barbiturates.
- Sulphonamides.
- Carbamazepine.
- Codeine.
- Penicillin.
- Phenytoin.

Angio-oedema

- Penicillin.
- Aspirin.
- Essential oils.

Gingival hyperplasia

- Phenytoin.
- Cyclosporin A.

- Nifedipine.
- Contraceptive pill.

Oral pigmentation

- ACTH (adrenocorticotropic hormone).
- Anticonvulsants.
- Busulphan.
- Contraceptive pill.

Lichenoid reactions

- Antiparkinsonian.
- Antiarrythmics.
- Antidiuretics.
- Beta-blockers.
- Antihypertensives.

Pemphigus-like reactions

- Penicillamine.
- Rifampicin.

Pemphigoid-like reactions

- Frusemide.
- Clonidine.

Salivary glands

Swelling

- Insulin.
- Methyldopa.
- Sulphonamides.
- Chlorhexidine.

Pain

- Cytotoxics.
- Methyldopa.

Ptyalism

- Anticholinesterases.
- Ketamine.
- Mercurials.

Xerostomia

- Atropine.
- Tricyclic antidepressants.
- MAOIs (mono-amine oxidase inhibitors).
- Antihistamines.
- Phenothiazine.

Disturbed taste

- Antithyroids.
- Lithium.
- Metronidazole.
- Penicillamine.

Blood values

Table 3.2   Blood values.

Test	Values	Importance
Haemoglobin Hb	♀ 11.5–16.5 g/100 ml	↓ in anaemia
	♂ 13–18 g/100 ml	
– Women	< 11.5 g/dL	
– Men	< 13.5 g/dL	
Haemotocrit or PCV	♀ 37–47%	↓ in anaemia
	♂ 40–54%	
RBC count	♀ 4.2–5.4 10^{12}/litre	↓ in anaemia
	♂ 4.2–6.1 10^{12}/litre	↑ in polycythemia
MCV = $\dfrac{PCV}{RBC}$	78–99 fl	↑ in B_{12} or folate deficiency & liver disease ↓ in iron deficiency
MCH = $\dfrac{Hb}{RBC}$	27–31 pg	↓ in anaemia ↑ in pernicious anaemia
WBC count	4–10 10^9/litre	↓ in leukaemia/ infection/ pregnancy
Platelets	150–400 10^9/litre	↓ related to leukaemia, drugs infections, autoimmune
ESR	0–15 mmh	↑ in temporal arteritis/infection/ pregnancy
Bleeding time (Duke)	1–3 min	
Coagulation time (Lee and White)	3–8 min	

Use an EDTA tube except for ESR test which requires a citrated tube.
ESR = erythrocyte sedimentation rate.
MCH = mean cell haemoglobin.
MCV = mean cell volume.
PCV = packed cell volume.
RBC = red blood cells.
WBC = white blood cells.

High-risk patients

Hepatitis B immunisation

High-risk groups

- IV drug abusers.
- Homosexuals and prostitutes.
- Haemophiliacs.
- Renal dialysis patients.
- Immunosuppressed transplant patients.
- Institutionalised patients.
- Recent history of jaundice.
- Immigrants from south-east Asia/Africa.
- Consorts with all the above.

Procedure if hepatitis B carrier is suspected

1 Contact general medical practitioner (GMP) for update of medical information.
2 Refer to hospital for viral tests prior to commencement of extensive dental treatment.
3 Emergency pain-relief procedures may be carried out but with full precautions if antigenic status is unknown.

Interpretation of serological markers of hepatitis B

1 HBsAg – infective risk.
2 HbeAg – high infective risk.
3 HbcAg – post/present infective.
4 BHsAb – immunity.
5 HBeAb – no special risk.
6 DNA polymerase – used to monitor disease progression.

Prevention of cross-infection

Planning
- Make appointment last of day.
- Ensure nursing staff have been immunised against hepatitis B.

Setting up
- Protective clothing:
  - disposable rubber gloves
  - face masks
  - gowns
  - eye shields.
- All instruments should be either autoclavable or disposable.
- Set out minimum of equipment necessary.
- Rigid burn bin to collect sharps.
- Two stout plastic bags to receive non-sharp disposables.
- Disposable metal foil dish for use as spittoon.
- Portable suction system.
- Plastic bag coverage over x-ray machine over handset controls.
- Prepare any intra-oral radiographs each in separate sealable plastic envelopes.
- Have available 2% glutaraldehyde solution and sodium hypochlorite solution (1 in 10 dilution household bleach).

Treatment procedures
1 Plan treatment for a minimum of visits.
2 Use slow handpiece, scale by hand, avoid three-in-one syringe, ultrasonic instruments or air turbines.
3 Use silicone impression materials. Place these in 2% glutaraldehyde for one hour, rinse and place in a fresh solution for a further three hours. Transport to laboratory labelled as 'danger of infection'.

4 To avoid needle-stick injuries, needles should not be recapped, bent, broken or removed from disposable syringes.

Clearing away

1 Place all sharps in burn bin.
2 Wearing operating gloves, transfer non-disposable instruments uncleaned to the autoclave and sterilise immediately.
3 Place all non-sharp disposables into the ready-for-use plastic bags.
4 Remove operating gloves and place in the same bags.
5 Wash carefully in Hibiscrub.
6 Wearing heavy-duty rubber gloves, remove instruments from steriliser. Clean instruments in detergent and warm water and re-sterilise.
7 All non-disposable items which cannot be autoclaved should be soaked in 2% glutaraldehyde for one hour, washed in detergent then left to soak in a fresh solution for a further ten hours (e.g. overnight).
8 Still wearing rubber gloves (above) wipe all surfaces: metallic surfaces 2% glutaraldehyde, non-metallic surfaces sodium hypochlorite. Rinse and dry surfaces with alcohol.
9 Remove gloves, seal burn bin and plastic bags. Check that they are labelled, in accordance with the code of practice, 'danger of infection'.

Accidental spillage of blood or pus

1 Drop paper tissue onto surface.
2 Gently flood with 10% solution of available chlorine (Domestos) for at least ten minutes.
3 Wearing heavy rubber gloves wash area with detergent and water then dry thoroughly.

Procedure in the event of needle-stick injury

1 Discard needle into sharps bin.
2 Encourage bleeding.
3 Wash thoroughly.
4 Record full details in accident book.
5 Further action depends on immunity:
   a if covered, no further action
   b not immune, requires hyperimmune antiserum within 12 hours
   c questionable immunity, check antibody levels.
6 Should an exposure of this type result in an illness then it will need to be reported formally by the employer to the Health and Safety Executive under the Health and Safety Regulations (1985) The Reporting of Injuries, Disease and Dangerous Occurrences (RIDDOR).

Section 3

4 Orthodontics in general practice

Introduction

Most orthodontic patients are treated in the early permanent dentition, typically at 12–13 years old when the second molars erupt. However, it is important to make an annual assessment in the mixed dentition to identify developing problems and where necessary arrange treatment. Early intervention can simplify or eliminate the need for later treatment. A guide to dental milestones and eruption dates is included for reference later in the chapter.

Mixed dentition

The most common problems or conditions to look for in the mixed dentition are: premature loss of deciduous molars, retained deciduous teeth, submerging molars, impacted first permanent molars, supernumerary teeth, digit habits, median diastema, first permanent molars of poor prognosis and cross-bites.

It is wise to palpate for permanent maxillary canines in the labial sulcus at the age of 9–10 years; it is widely accepted that early removal of deciduous canines can avoid palatal impaction at a later date. There are some simple procedures with removable or simple fixed appliances that can be carried out in the practice at this stage, e.g. correction of anterior or posterior cross-bite and space maintenance.

Permanent dentition

Unless you are particularly experienced with modern orthodontic therapy it is always best to take advice from a specialist. Remember that even though you may not carry out the work you will be asked to participate in the treatment plan. This might include tooth extraction, supervision of dental health throughout appliance therapy, re-enforcement of the retention regime and at times it may be necessary to carry out emergency repairs to appliances.

Tooth development milestones

Primary dentition eruption

See Table 4.1.

Secondary dentition calcification

- First molars   Birth
- Incisors and canines   3 to 5 months
- Lower lateral incisors   3 to 4 months
- Upper lateral incisors   10 to 12 months
- First premolars   1.5 to 2 years
- Second premolars and molars   2 to 3 years
- Third molars   7 to 10 years

Secondary dentition eruption

See Table 4.2.

Table 4.1   Primary dentition eruption.

Age (months)	6	9	12	18	24
	A	B	C	D	E

Table 4.2   Secondary dentition eruption.

Age (years)	6	7	8	9	10	11	12	> 17
Maxillary	6	1	2	–	4	3 and 5	7	8
Mandibular	6 and 1	2	–	3	4	5	7	8

Dental milestones

- Birth: deciduous incisors and canines half-formed/deciduous molars initial calcification/first molar cusp tips calcified.
- 3 years: eciduous dentition fully erupted/permanent incisor and first molar crowns complete/canines half-formed/premolar and second molar cusp tips calcified.
- 6 years: first molars and lower central incisors erupt/other crowns well formed.
- 8 years: second molar crowns formed.
- 9 years: check position of maxillary canines – radiograph if necessary.
- 11 years: assess orthodontic situation/assess submerged deciduous molars.

Patient assessment

The following is a guide to what to look for when making an assessment. Study models and appropriate radiographs are essential when making a definitive diagnosis.

Case history

- Patient/parental concerns.
- Social history.
- Relevant dental or orthodontic history (trauma, early loss, digit sucking, musical instrument play).
- Relevant medical history.

Extra-oral

- Skeletal:
  - anteroposterior – Class I, II or III
  - vertical – long/short/normal face (face height)
  - lateral – facial asymmetry
  - TMJ dysfunction – check for signs and symptoms.
- Soft tissues
  - lips – competent/incompetent, form and tonicity, upper lip length and relationship of lower lip to upper incisors
  - facial profile – concave/convex/normal and nasolabial angle
  - tongue position – look for position at rest and in rare circumstances a tongue thrust
  - digit-sucking habits.

Intra-oral

- Teeth present:
  - 87654321 12345678
  - 87654321 12345678.

- Dental health:
  - oral hygiene
  - existing restorations
  - caries
  - hypoplasia/mottling/staining
  - trauma – evidence of previous trauma.
- Lower arch:
  - crowding
  - missing teeth
  - impacted teeth
  - incisor inclinations
  - rotations.
- Upper arch:
  - ditto.
- Arch relations:
  - incisors – Class I, Class II Div I, Class II Div II, Class III
  - molars – Class I, II or III
  - overjet
  - overbite
  - centre-line shift
  - cross-bites – anterior and/or posterior, with/without displacement.

Radiographic assessment

An OPG (orthopantomography) is a useful screening radiograph for a preliminary assessment. In addition a standard occlusal view or periapical may be needed if there is a history of trauma, missing teeth, or where the presence of supernumeraries may be suspected.

Treatment summary

This helps to collate your thoughts on the main features of the malocclusion and will help with treatment planning, e.g. nine-year-old boy with a developing Class II Div I, OJ 8 mm already with trauma to upper left central incisor. Possible candidate for early advice and treatment.

Treatment plan (options)

- Observe.
- Refer to specialist.
- Proceed with active treatment e.g. extractions and/or simple URA (upper removable appliance).

Orthodontic indices

There are two orthodontic indices widely in use throughout the UK. You should familiarise yourself with both indices: the Index of Treatment Need (IOTN) and the Peer Assessment Rating (PAR).

Index of Treatment Need (IOTN)

This is used to prioritise orthodontic treatment on the basis of severity of malocclusion and need for treatment. There are five categories ranging from 1 to 5. Currently NHS orthodontists can accept patients classified as IOTN 4 to 5. Patients in categories 2 to 3 are often referred by practitioners but may not be eligible to NHS orthodontic treatment.

Table 4.3 shows more details for IOTN.

Table 4.3   Index of treatment needed.

	Overjet	Reverse overjet	Anterior or posterior crossbites	Displacement of teeth	Anterior or posterior open bite	Overbite	Other
Grade 5 Very great	Increased greater than 9 mm	Greater than 3.5 mm with masticatory or speech impairment		Submerged deciduous teeth			Extensive hypodontia with restorative implication Impeded eruption of teeth due to crowding, pathology Cleft lip or palate
Grade 4 Great	Increased 6.1–9 mm	Greater than 3.5 mm with no masticatory or speech impairment	Greater than 2 mm between RCP and ICP	Severe greater than 4 mm	Extreme greater than 4 mm	Increased and complete with gingival trauma	Hypodontia Posterior lingual cross bites with no functional occlusion Impacted, tipped supplemental teeth
Grade 3 Moderate	Increased 3.6–6 mm	1.1–3.5 mm	1.1–2 mm discrepancy	2.1–4 mm	2.1–4 mm	Increased and complete without gingival trauma	
Grade 2	Increased 3.6–6 mm	0.1–1 mm	Up to 1 mm discrepancy between RCP and ICP	1.1–2 mm	1.1–2 mm	3.5 mm or more without gingival contact	Can include up to half a unit discrepancy
Grade 1 None	Minor malocclusions or displacement less than 1 mm						

IOTN is accompanied by an aesthetic index (SCAN) based on appearance of the teeth.

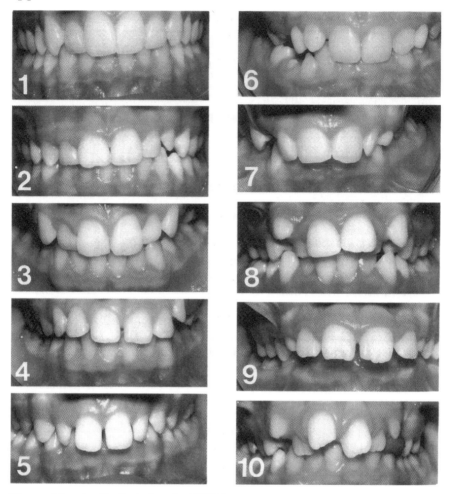

Figure 4.1   Aesthetic index for IOTN.

Peer Assessment Rating (PAR)

This is used to assess treatment standards. Scores are recorded for a number of occlusal features from before and after study models. The difference between the scores can be calculated and expressed as a percentage change in PAR. A score of 70% and above is considered a high standard and 30% and below no appreciable difference. It is important to note that the higher the PAR score at the beginning the more severe the malocclusion, and if you start with a low score it will be difficult to achieve a significant reduction.

Referring a patient to a specialist

All referral letters should be concise, relevant and polite. If radiographs and study models are available they should be included with the letter. In all cases the following information is required.

1   Name, title and address of person to whom you are referring the patient.
2   Patient's name, address and date of birth.
3   Reason for referral.
4   Request for advice and/or treatment.
5   Any previous orthodontic treatment with dates.
6   Relevant medical/social history.
7   Diagnosis.
8   Patient's attitude.

Appliance design and prescription

You should use a standard laboratory prescription form and it is important that you design the appliance yourself. You should specify the main features of retention (e.g. Adams cribs), active components (e.g. mid-line screws and springs) and baseplate design (e.g. coverage of baseplate and biteplanes when required). Use the wire gauge guide in Table 4.4 to specify the wire needed for each component.

Table 4.4   Wire gauge guide.

Gauge	Usage
0.4	Z-spring for lateral incisors
0.5	Finger spring
	Z-spring
	T-spring
	Stop (hard stainless steel wire)
	Roberts Retractor with tubing
	Supported buccal canine retractor
0.6	Adams crib on deciduous canines
0.7	Adams crib
	Southend clasp
	Fitted labial bow
	U-loop buccal canine retractor
	Adams buccal canine retractor
	Stop (soft stainless steel wire)
0.8	Split labial bow
	U-loop labial bow
	Adams crib with buccal tube
0.9	Labial bow – Andresen
	High labial bow
1.25	Coffin spring
	Whisker bow – inner
1.5	Whisker bow – outer
	Incisal cleat ($\times$ 0.8 mm half round)

Further reading

- Mitchell L (1998) *An Introduction to Orthodontics*. Oxford University Press, Oxford.
- Shaw WC, O'Brien KD and Richmond S (1991) Quality control in orthodontics: indices of treatment need and treatment standards. *BDJ*. **170**: 107–12.

Websites

- British Orthodontic Society (BOS): www.bos.org.uk/.
- Dental Practice Board (DPB): www.dpb.nhs.uk/.

Section 4

5 Prescribing in practice

Responsibilities

- To prescribe with appropriate treatment where clinically justified, with patient advice.
- To be aware of rules and regulations associated with prescription, storage and dispensing, either NHS or private.
- To be familiar (with other members of your team) with standard resuscitation procedures and management of common medical emergencies which may arise in dental practice.
- To report any suspected adverse reaction to drugs/materials.

Practical prescribing in practice

- Know your pharmacology and have an up-to-date reference book available in the practice.
- From September 2004 the Dental Practitioners' Formulary (DPF) has been integrated into the British National Formulary (BNF). This must be readily available in the surgery.

In the body of the BNF numerous side headings facilitate the identification of advice on oral conditions. Preparations that may be prescribed on NHS dental prescriptions are picked out under appropriate preparation entries.

You must make yourself familiar with the first sections of the BNF including: how to use the BNF, changes for that edition, guidance on prescribing especially prescription writing, controlled drugs, adverse reactions, prescribing for children, the elderly and prescribing in dental practice.

Also be familiar with the Appendixes and DPF lists.

Read the data sheets published by drug companies and supplied with medicines, read MIMS and make sure you have taken account of this information before issuing a prescription either by hand or computer.

Essential information

1   Name and address of prescriber.
2   Name and address of patient.
3   Date of birth. Child's age in years and months.
4   The preparation – official name (e.g. ampicillin).

   NB: the proprietary name limits the pharmacist to a specific product; the generic drug name allows the pharmacist to provide the most convenient product.

5   Form (tablets, capsules, etc.).
6   Dosage and total quantity to be dispensed.
7   Prescriber's signature.

   Prescribe where only clinically justified. There is a rising concern about humans' increasing resistance to antibiotics and various levels of allergic responses.

   Note: Some preparations are cheaper than the prescription charge if bought over the counter.

- Formulary essential for drug information.
- Abbreviations not essential but useful:
  - Bd: twice a day
  - Tds: three times each day
  - Qds/qid: four times each day
  - Nocte: at night
  - Prn: as required
  - Ql: as much as desired
  - Qh: hourly.

Misuse of Drugs Regulations Act 1974

- Replaces the DDA: Dangerous Drugs Act.
- Controls the prescribing of addictive drugs.
- Dental surgeon can keep in stock, administer or prescribe controlled drugs only if genuinely needed for dental purposes.
- Important drugs of addiction are:
  - opiates – including morphine derivatives
  - stimulants of the central nervous system – cocaine and amphetamines.

Controlled drugs are divided into three classes:

- Class A – addictive and harmful.
- Class B – oral amphetamines, cannabis, codeine.
- Class C – related to amphetamines.

Prescribing controlled drugs

- The address of the prescriber must be in the UK.
- The pharmacist must be familiar with the signature of the prescriber.

- Drug must not be dispensed after 13 weeks of the prescription date.
- The entire prescription must be in the handwriting of the prescriber and in ink.
- Must show:
  - the prescriber's name
  - patient's name and address
  - form of preparations
  - strength of preparation
  - total quantity in both words and figures
  - prescription must be endorsed for dental treatment only.

  For dental treatment only:
  - usual signature of prescriber
  - date.

Private prescribing

A prescription may be written on any form of paper (not NHS FP14 form). The prescriber's name and address must be clearly visible. Same rules apply as above, only the patient will have to pay the full amount.

Private/NHS interface

While everybody is entitled to NHS treatment and hence NHS prescription, you should not give private patients an NHS prescription associated with a private course of treatment. If giving an NHS prescription to a private patient for an occasional treatment course, make sure an NHS form is signed and kept in the patient's card, even if it is not submitted for payment, and indicate clearly on the records that no private fee was charged for that course of treatment.

It is wisest not to mix private treatment and NHS prescribing.

Referring

Responsibilities

The dentist has the responsibility of appropriate referral of a patient for a second opinion, advice and/or treatment when the patient's problem/treatment required is deemed by the dentist to be beyond the dentist's capabilities, experience or present facilities. That responsibility requires that the dentist refers to an appropriate person (specialist, special interest, qualified), with appropriate facilities and appropriate treatment regimes available (type of treatment and whether primary care, secondary care or private) and including interpractice referrals.

Any referral must be done with the informed consent of the patient.

The specialist/referral dentist

The specialist/referral dentist has the responsibility of only doing treatment appropriate to the referral with the appropriate explanations, informed consent (including timings and any costs), access to continuing and emergency care and communications with the referring dentist.

Referring letter

Ideally proformas should exist in the practice protocols which have been agreed with the specialist services being used and are available either as electronic or as hard copies.

Following are two examples of referral templates for period-ontal treatment to a periodontal specialist.

The Dental Practice
Address

Referred by

Request for Periodontal Consultation   Date _____

Patient details: Mr Mrs Miss Ms   (please circle)   DOB _____

Surname: _____

First Names: _____   Tel. (home) _____

Address:_____   (work) _____

_____

Referring dentist: _____   Relevant MH _____

Reason for referral: _____

Please give (where available) last 3 BPE chartings with dates:

—/—/— date_____   —/—/—/ date_____   —/—/— date_____

Please indicate the following on a scale 0–3 (0 = none, 3 = gross):

Plaque [ ]   Calculus [ ]   Gingival inflammation [ ]

Has the patient had an acute periodontal problem in the last 5 years? If yes, please give brief details:

_____

Please give the frequency with which the patient visits the hygienist:

3 montly [ ] 6 montly [ ] Yearly [ ] Not applicable [ ] Other (please specify)_____

If the dentist has been carrying out the periodontal treatment please indicate no. of visits per year _____

Has the patient evern seen a Specialist Periodontist? If so please give brief details:_____

_____

Please indicate which radiographs are available and dates:

_____

Please include relevant radiographs that may aid diagnosis (these will be returned).

Specialist Periodontal Treatment Referral Form

Patient's Name: .... DOB ....

Address:.. Tel. No.. .... (Work)

.... (Home)

Postcode: .... Date of Referral: ....

Provisional diagnosis: .... Plaque index score: ....

Does the patient smoke?   YES ☐   NO ☐

CPITN/BPE score ☐☐
                 ☐☐

Date of last radiographs ....

Radiographs enclosed   YES ☐   NO ☐
All radiographs will be returned

Medical History including medication: ....

....

Details of previous periodontal therapy with dates: ....

....

....

Outcome: ....

....

Please provide:
 • Advice and treatment plan only   YES ☐   NO ☐
 • Treatment as appropriate   YES ☐   NO ☐

Dentist's signature .... Date ....

Name .... Tel: ....

Practice Address: ....

....

....

The vocational dental practitioner (VDP) should be made familiar with these at induction and hopefully during the vocational training (VT) year will be able to visit many of the referral services used.

Information to be included in referring letter proforma

- Keep concise and polite.
- Practice address and contact phone number.
- Patient name, address, phone number, sex and date of birth.
- Patient medical history and if possible doctor's name and address.
- About patient and relevant dental history.
- About complaint and duration, signs and symptoms.
- Specific request for treatment or advice, second opinion.
- Patient attitude towards or understanding of the problem and their consent for referral.
- Urgency of referral and any treatment.
- NHS/private.
- Referring dentist's name typed and signed
- Enclosures – radiograph, pictures, mouth maps.

It is helpful if specific proformas are agreed with each specialist and exist electronically in practice computer systems.

Dos and don'ts and helpful hints

- Get to know the people you are referring to during the year, preferably visiting them.
- Practice referral list and proformas.
- Be aware of any time targets (since December 2000 head and

neck cancer maximum two weeks to be seen) and any fast-track protocols.

- Likewise be aware of prioritisation pathways used – urgency/ patients in pain.
- NHS/private interface – if no NHS provision inform PCT and check out of area/referral possibilities.
- Intra-practice referrals and shared appointments.
- Informing other professionals treating same patients e.g. doctor, orthodontist.

Section 5

6 Pain, trauma and emergencies

Differential diagnosis of toothache

See Table 6.1.

Trauma and avulsion

When a patient presents following a traumatic dental injury, a thorough dental and medical history and examination must be taken.

Trauma record

Personal details

- Name.
- Address.
- Date of birth.

Medical history

- Congenital heart disease or severe immunosuppression; contraindications for prolonged endodontic treatment.

Table 6.1 Differential diagnosis of toothache.

	Is pain spontaneous?	Is pain continuous?	Is pain well located?	Is tooth TTP?	Soft tissue tenderness?	Is tooth vital?	Any radiographic changes?	Other relevant signs?
A. Common Causes								
1. Origin – Tooth:								
Reversible acute pulpitis	X	To stimulus	X	X	X	✓	X	
Irreversible acute pulpitis	X/✓	X	X	X	X	X/✓	X	
Dentinal hypersensitivity	X	To stimulus	✓	X	X	✓	X	Exposed dentine
Chronic pulpitis	✓	Occasional	X	X	X	X	X	
Acute apical periodontitis	✓	✓	✓	Slightly	Possibly	X	Possible periapical widening	? Sinus
Chronic apical periodontitis	✓	Occasional	✓	Slightly	Possibly	X	Possible periapical widening	? Sinus
Acute apical abscess	✓	✓	✓	✓	✓	X	Periapical radiolucency	Lymphadenopathy
2. Origin – Gingival/supporting tissues:								
Lateral periodontal abscess	✓	✓	✓	✓	Possibly	✓	Periodontal bone loss	Periodontal pocketing
Acute ulcerative gingivitis		Soreness	✓	X	✓	✓	Possibly bony cratering	Destruction of inter-dental papillae
Pericoronitis	✓		✓	X	✓	✓	Possibly follicle around tooth	Presence of partially erupted tooth

NOTE 1. The above table only applies if source of pain is not multifactorial e.g.: Endo-perio lesions would present with a combination of the above.
2. Vitality Test results can be highly variable, especially in heavily restored and/or multi-rooted teeth.

B. Less Common Causes (which must be considered if local factors are eliminated).

Referred pain from: Maxillary sinus infections and neoplasms.
  Salivary gland infections and neoplasms.
  Vascular system e.g. migraines.
  Ear infections and neoplasma.
  TMJ/Muscles of mastication; especially myofacial pain dysfunction/bruxism.
  Nervous system e.g. neuralgias.

TTP = tender to percussion.

- Bleeding disorders.
- Allergies.
- Tetanus immunisation status. Soil contamination of wound will require referral for tetanus toxoid injection if no booster in last five years.

History of traumatic injury

- *When?* The time interval between injury and treatment can significantly affect the treatment and prognosis.
- *Where?* Tetanus cover may be required.
- *How?* Non-accidental injury (NAI) may be suspected if discrepancy between history and clinical findings.
- *Lost teeth/tooth fragments* been accounted for? (Consider soft tissue and/or chest x-rays especially if there has been loss of consciousness.)
- *Other symptoms?* Loss of consciousness, concussion, headache, vomiting or amnesia. Hospital referral for further investigation indicated.
- *Treatment already received?*
- *Previous dental history?* Previous trauma could affect diagnostic tests or indicate an accident-prone child or NAI.

Examination

Extra-oral
- General state of patient. Look for signs of shock and concussion.
- Bruising.
- Facial lacerations.
- Bone fractures.
- Mandibular movement. Check for dislocation or fracture.

Intra-oral

- Soft tissue lacerations. Check for foreign bodies in soft tissues.
- Tooth fractures: classification.
- Alveolar fractures.
- Tooth fractures/displacement/mobility classification?
- Tooth colour.
- Check for foreign bodies in soft tissues.
- Sensitivity tests.
- Reaction to percussion.

Radiographic examination

- Periapical film.
- Occlusal film.
- Dental panoramic tomograph.

Other considerations

- Treatment planning.
- Refer on to oral surgery department/casualty.
- Tetanus cover required?
- Photographs.

The avulsed tooth

Immediate action by patient

1   Replace tooth in socket.
2   a   Hold tooth only by crown, rinse root gently in cold tap water.

   b   Replace the tooth in the socket or store tooth in milk – do
       not allow to dry out.
   c   If tooth replaced bite gently on a handkerchief to keep it
       in place.
3 Visit dentist as soon as possible.

Immediate action by dentist

1 If tooth has been replanted skip to step 'f'.
2 If tooth in milk:
   a   Wash in sterile normal saline.
   b   Check socket for fracture/foreign body.
   c   Irrigate socket with normal saline to remove clot and
       foreign material.
   d   Measure length of tooth and assess root development.
   e   Replace tooth gently but firmly in socket.
   f   Splint for 7–10 days with functional splint.
   g   Check occlusion.
   h   Take baseline radiograph.
   i   Give five-day course of antibiotics.

NB: If tooth out of mouth for less than 30 minutes, follow a to e
as above.
   If tooth out of mouth for more than 30 minutes rehydrate in
normal saline for five minutes, then follow a to f above.

Follow-up by dentist

Closed apex
1 Extirpate pulp within first week of replantation.
2 Intracanal dressing antibiotic/steroid paste (Ledermix).

3 Subsequent intracanal dressings non-setting calcium hydroxide changed at three-monthly intervals.
4 Definitive root-canal treatment at 12 months.

Open apex

- May revascularise if out of the mouth for less than 45 minutes.
- Radiograph regularly to check for:
  - normal root development
  - signs of resorption
  - apical pathology.
- If out of mouth for more than 45 minutes treat as for closed apex but continue with calcium hydroxide until apical barrier forms (max. 2–3 years).
- NB: Must have long-term treatment plan in the event of loss of tooth.

Teeth with dry storage time of more than one hour

1 Place tooth in 2.4% sodium fluoride solution for 20 minutes.
2 Root fill at chair side.
3 Replant and splint rigidly for six weeks.

This treatment will produce ankylosis allowing the tooth to be retained as a natural space maintainer.

Splinting times

Subluxation: splint for 7 days only if significantly tender to percussion (TTP)
Avulsion: 7–10 days functional splinting.
Displacement injuries: 2–3 weeks functional splinting.

Root fracture: 2–3 weeks functional splinting.
Dentoalveolar fractures: 3–4 weeks rigid splinting
NB: Review current research for update.

Non-accidental injury (NAI)

- Some 50% of NAI cases have extra and intra-oral facial trauma.
- Investigation requires considerable tact and experience and should be left to those suitably qualified.
- If the child is in no immediate danger consult their GP who may be aware of a family history.
- Consult your local authority policy document on child abuse.
- Subsequent liaison with the hospital is important such that follow up can be made in the event of non-attendance.
- Advice can also be sought from the social services and from the National Society for the Prevention of Cruelty to Children (NSPCC).
- Seek advice from your defence union.
- Ensure that all records are accurate and contemporaneous.

See Figures 6.1–6.5 as guides for assessment of fractured and displaced deciduous and adult teeth.

History

1 Inadequate explanation of injury and delay in seeking medical advice for injuries.
2 Frequent visits for medical advice – possibly a cry for help.
3 Known or suspected previous child abuse.
4 Inappropriate or disturbed parental behaviour.

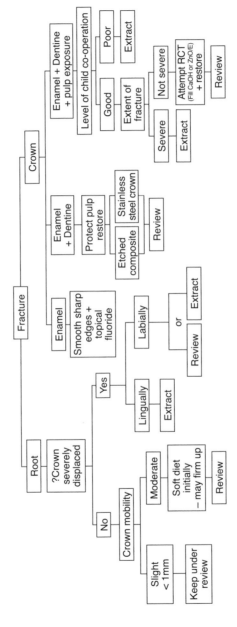

Figure 6.1 Assessment and treatment of fractured primary anterior teeth.

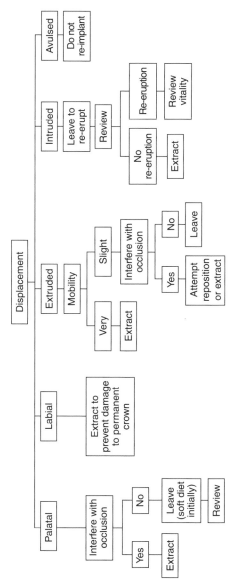

Figure 6.2 Assessment and treatment of displaced primary anterior teeth.

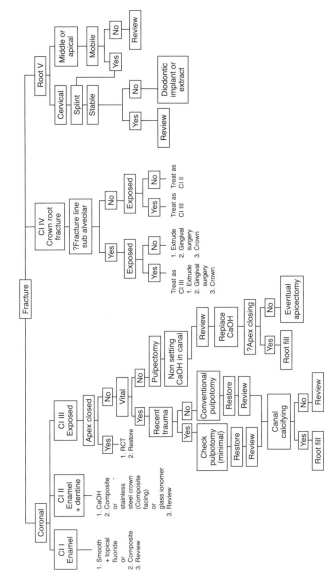

Figure 6.3   Assessment and treatment of fractured permanent anterior teeth.

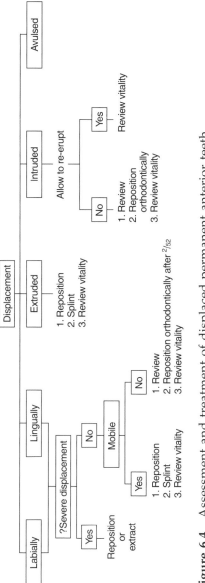

Figure 6.4   Assessment and treatment of displaced permanent anterior teeth.

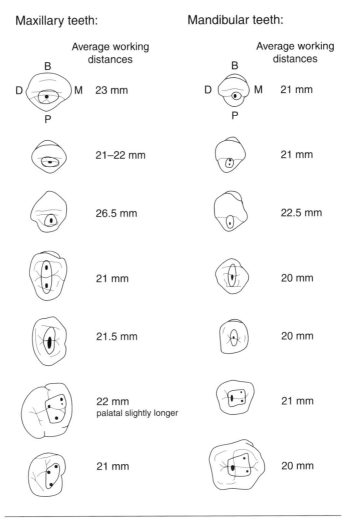

Maxillary teeth:

Average working distances

23 mm

21–22 mm

26.5 mm

21 mm

21.5 mm

22 mm
palatal slightly longer

21 mm

Mandibular teeth:

Average working distances

21 mm

21 mm

22.5 mm

20 mm

20 mm

21 mm

20 mm

Points to remember:

4; 74% have >1 canal with >1 foramen.
5; 75% have 1 canal with 1 foramen.
6,7; assume these teeth have 4 canals (2MB, 1P, 1DB) until second MB canal cannot be found.
1,2; >40% have 2 canals but separate foramina are seen in only 1%.
4,5; may have 2 canals, but these usually re-join to give 1 foramen.
6,7; generally have 3 canals (MB, ML, D) but 33% have 4 canals.

References:
Pitt T. R. (1997) *Harty's Endodontics in Clinical Practice*. Butterworth-Heinemann, Oxford.
Mitchell L, Mitchell D.A. (2005) *Oxford Handbook of Clinical Dentistry (3e)*. Oxford University Press, Oxford.

Figure 6.5   Access cavities for root canal therapy.

Table 6.2 Acute Medical Conditions. Symptoms and signs.

	Pain	Pupils	Breathing	Pulse	Skin	Consciousness level	Others	Treatment (Drugs and actions taken)
Anaphylaxis			Wheeze	Weak & Rapid	Cold, Clammy, Itch, Pallor	Loss	Oedema	(i) Adrenalin 1 ml of 1:1000 i.m. or s.c., then (ii) Hydrocortisone 200 mg i.v., then (iii) Chlorpheniramine 10–20 mg i.v. slowly
Angina	Retrosternal		?Laboured	Regular				GTN sublingually 0.5 mg
Asthma			Wheeze Dyspnoea		Cyanosis if severe			Normal bronchodilator, Oxygen, Hydrocortisone 200 mg i.m./i.v.
Cardiac arrest		?Dilated	Absent	Absent	Cyanosis Cold	Loss		(i) Call for ambulance with defibrillator (ii) Initiate CPR until help arrives or conscious level restored (iii) Defibrillation
CVA (Stroke)						Transient Loss	Hemiplegia	(i) Call for ambulance, monitor breathing circulation (ii) Secure airway, commence CPR if required
Corticosteroid insufficiency				Weak & Rapid	Pallor	Loss		400 mg Hydrocortisone i.v.
Epilepsy						Loss	Jerking Incontinence Vomiting	(i) Secure airway (ii) Lay patient away from harm (iii) If status epilepticus ensures, 10 mg Diazepam i.v. or i.m.
Faint		Dilation		Slow	Cold & Clammy Pallor	Transient Loss	Dizzy Weakness Nausea	(i) Lay patient flat (ii) Secure airway (iii) Loosen tight clothing (iv) Glucose drink
Hypoglycaemia				Rapid	Warm & Clammy	Loss	Dizzy Disorientation	If conscious, sweet drink If unconscious 60 ml of 50% glucose i.v., or 1 mg glucagon injected by any route
Myocardial infarction	Severe Retrosternal		Dyspnoea	Irregular		Loss		(i) Seek medical assistance (ii) Oxygen (iii) Warmth and reassurance (iv) GTN sublingually (v) Monitor vital signs

CPR = cardiopulmonary resuscitation; GTN = glyceryl trinitrate; CVA = cerebral vascular accident.

Signs

Psychological

1 Silent hyperalertness, an inhibition of natural behaviour. 'Frozen awareness.' Tense rigidity in adult presence.
2 Behavioural activity may range from hyperactive 'naughtiness' to withdrawn apathy.
3 Many show demanding, 'clingy' behaviour in an attempt to gain greater mothering.

Physical

1 Skin injuries present in over 90% of cases, but neglect and deprivation can occur without other signs of maltreatment.
2 Height, weight, cleanliness, general care and clothing.
3 Lesions of various vintages.
4 Location of injuries – accidental bruising tends to be random in both size and shape and located over bony prominences such as shins, knees, forehead, etc.
5 Some of the more common characteristic injuries are listed below:
   - fingertip bruising, commonly on face
   - facial squeezing
   - grip marks, pinch marks, bites and cigarette burns
   - frenum tearing
   - signs of violent bottle feeding
   - petechial haemorrhage on ear lobes (blue spotted ear)
   - bilateral black eyes
   - other bodily injuries such as immersion scalds.

Remember to seek advice. Aggressive questioning of parents and involvement of the police is counterproductive.

Emergencies: the basic procedure

1   Faint.
2   Hypoglycaemia.
3   Cardiac emergencies.
4   Epilepsy.
5   Corticosteroid insufficiency.
6   Asthma.
7   Anaphylaxis.
8   Hysteria.
9   Haemorrhage.

Faint

Clinical features

- Moist, cold skin, dilated pupils, muscular twitching.
- Pallor.
- Dizziness, weakness, nausea and vomiting.
- Weak, slow pulse.

Management

- Lay patient as flat as is reasonably comfortable and, in the absence of breathlessness, raise legs to improve cerebral circulation.
- Loosen clothing.
- Glucose drink may be useful.
- Consider other causes if recovery not rapid.

Hypoglycaemia

Clinical features

- Moist, warm skin.
- Dizziness and disorientation, difficulty concentrating.
- Full, rapid pulse, change in behaviour.
- Hunger.

Management

- Lay patient flat.
- Glucose orally if conscious
- If unconscious glucagon 1 mg (1 unit) given by intramuscular (or subcutaneous) injection. Half this dose for a child under eight years or under 25 kg body weight.
- If the glucagon is ineffective or contraindicated, up to 50 ml of glucose IV infusion 20%. Alternatively 25 ml of glucose intravenous infusion 50%, but this is very viscous and difficult to administer.
- Summon medical assistance.

Cardiac emergencies

Clinical features

- Crushing pain across front of chest, which may radiate towards shoulder and down arm, or into neck and jaw.
- Breathlessness.
- Nausea/vomiting
- Weak pulse, may become unconscious.

Management

- Reassure patient and loosen any tight clothing.
- Give GTN (glyceryl trinitrate) spray or tablets sublingually.
- If no improvement summon medical assistance.
- Place patient in the position that is most comfortable for them; in the presence of breathlessness this will be sitting upright.
- Provide oxygen (50% nitrous oxide and 50% oxygen if available).
- Give a single dose of aspirin (150–300 mg).
- If the patient collapses and loses consciousness start standard resuscitation procedures.

Epilepsy

Clinical features

- Sudden loss of consciousness.
- Repetitive jerking movements.
- Occasional incontinence and vomiting.
- Recovery may be slow; patient may remain confused for some time.

Management

- Do not attempt to restrain convulsive movements.
- After movements have stopped place patient in recovery position.
- Maintain airway.
- If not recovered after five minutes, give 10 mg diazepam intravenously (if possible) or intramuscularly.
- Consider medical attention for convulsions which are atypical, prolonged or if injury occurred.

Corticosteroid insufficiency

Clinical features

- Usually in patients on long-term corticosteroid therapy and up to two years after its withdrawal.
- Loss of consciousness.
- Weak, rapid pulse.
- Falling blood pressure.
- Pallor.

Management

- Lay patient flat.
- Give 100 mg hydrocortisone succinate intravenously.
- Give oxygen.
- Summon medical assistance.

Asthma

Clinical features

- Paroxysmal wheezing.
- Dyspnoea.
- Rapid pulse.

Management

- Reassure patient.
- Patients should use their normal bronchodilator. If they do not have one with them give two puffs of salbutamol (in a spacer if necessary).

- If patient not responding or becoming tachycardic give oxygen and adrenaline IM (intramuscular) as for anaphylaxis.
- Do not lay flat.
- Summon medical assistance. If there is likely to be a delay for an hour hydrocortisone 200 mg IV may be given.

Anaphylaxis

Clinical features

- Paraesthesia, circum oral and swelling of face.
- Loss of consciousness.
- Cold, clammy skin, wheezing and difficulty breathing.
- Oedema/urticaria.
- Falling blood pressure.
- Weak, rapid pulse.
- Pallor.

Management

- Lay patient flat.
- Raise legs.
- Summon medical assistance.
- Intramuscular dose of 0.5 ml adrenaline 1:1000. This dose is repeated if necessary at five-minute intervals according to blood pressure, pulse and respiratory function.
- Give oxygen.

Hysteria

Clinical features

- Anxiety.
- Hyperventilation.
- Disturbed consciousness.
- Tetany or paraesthesia.

Management

- Reassure after excluding other causes.
- Loosen tight clothing.
- Manage hyperventilation by getting patient to exhale into a bag and inhale from this.

Haemorrhage

Causes

- Usually locally after traumatic extraction.
- Drug therapy – e.g. aspirin, warfarin, clopidigrel.
- Occasionally haemorrhagic disorder.

Management

- Reassure patient.
- Clean mouth and locate source.
- Place pack, leave for 15 minutes under pressure.
- Enquire into family history/medical history.
- Use haemostatic pack in socket and suture under LA.
- If bleeding is uncontrollable, refer to hospital.

Equipment and drugs required for managing emergencies

First-aid treatment in the dental surgery should aim at improving the patient's condition or at least preventing it becoming worse without causing any harm.

Equipment

The GDC guidance from *Maintaining Standards* states that training should include the use of emergency drugs and the practice of resuscitation in a simulated emergency. It is essential that all premises where dental treatment takes place have available and in working order:

1 equipment with appropriate attachments to provide intermittent positive pressure ventilation of the lungs and a portable source of oxygen together with emergency drugs
2 oral airways to maintain the natural airway
3 portable suction equipment, independent of a power supply.

There is currently no definitive list of emergency drugs to be stocked. Practitioners are referred to the list contained in the BNF for guidance:

- adrenaline injection 1:1000
- aspirin dispersible tablets 300 mg
- chlorpheniramine injection 10 mg/ml 1ml ampule
- diazepam injection 5 mg/ml, 2 ml ampules
- dextrose tablets or glucose drink
- glucagon injection 1 unit vial
- glucose intravenous infusion, glucose 20% (200 mg/ml), 500 ml pack *or* glucose 50% (500 mg/ml) 50 ml prefilled syringe

- glyceryl trinitrate tablets and/or sprays
- hydrocortisone injection, hydrocortisone 100 mg
- oxygen
- salbutamol aerosol inhalation, salbutamol 100 mg/metered inhalation
- salbutamol injection, salbutamol 500 micrograms/ml 1 ml ampule.

Training

- Attend regular (e.g. annual) training classes with *all* practice staff.
- Have regular training exercises in the practice.
- Maintain all equipment at all times and have readily available.

For adult basic life support, *see* Figure 6.6.

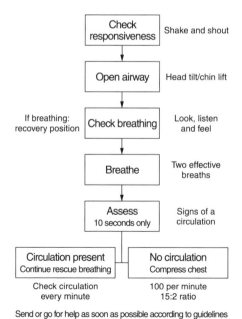

Figure 6.6   Adult basic life support from the Resuscitation Council UK.

Section 6

7 Oral cancer

Oral cancer screening

Oral cancer is one of the most debilitating and disfiguring of all malignancies. As a general dental practitioner (GDP), you are in the frontline of oral and dental care. It is your responsibility to prevent, diagnose and treat (or refer) dental and oral disease. You will manage this in two ways:

- reduction of risk through oral health education and
- identification and management of suspicious lesions.

Adopting a comprehensive screening policy, which is consistently applied and documented, allows early diagnosis and improves the patient's prognosis. Many patients with oral cancer are initially referred by their GDP.

Dental students can have variable experiences of the diagnosis and management of patient with head and neck malignancies.

If your knowledge needs reinforcing or updating at any stage of your career, information is easily available online from the BDA, and local maxillofacial units will often run teaching courses and clinics.

Why is oral cancer screening important?

Despite the fact that oral cancer has an incidence rate comparable with cervical cancer, there is little public awareness of mouth cancer. More surprisingly, although there have been major technological, medical and surgical advances in the treatment of oral cancer, the death rate for oral cancer now exceeds that for cervical cancer, with the crude five-year mortality rate being approximately 50%.

This has not significantly improved over the last 30 years, despite the fact that early diagnosis greatly improves the chance of complete cure. However, as a result of treatment for the disease, quality of life has been greatly improved. In the UK there are over 4300 new cases each year and over 1700 people will die from oral cancer.

Successful treatment of oral cancer relies on early detection of the disease. As a GDP providing primary dental care, it is your responsibility to regularly screen for oral cancer, in order to identify those patients who are at risk of developing oral cancer or have the early stages of the disease.

Who should be screened?

The FDI (World Dental Federation) states that a visual and digital palpation of the soft tissues should be part of *every* dental examination. Following this advice will ensure early detection of lesions in younger patients whose incidence of oral cancer is increasing, as well as patients in the traditionally acknowledged risk groups.

What are the risk factors for developing oral cancer?

Although the established risk factors for oral cancer are listed, you must be aware that the previous patterns of incidence no longer reflect the current situation (*see* Box 7.1).

Box 7.1 Oral cancer risk factors

Established risk factors:

- smoking tobacco
- chewing tobacco
- high alcohol consumption (synergistic with tobacco)
- presence of potentially malignant lesions and conditions
- previous oral/aerodigestive cancer
- sunlight exposure, age.

Passive smoking is also a risk factor not to be dismissed

Possible risk factors:

- dietary deficiency
- viral infections
- candida
- immune deficiency or suppression
- chronic sepsis in the mouth
- familial or genetic predisposition.

The cultural use of chewing tobacco is a specific concern. Among the Asian population, oral cancer is a major health risk; it causes 30% of cancer-related deaths within this group. The more recent introduction of Gutkha (sweetened tobacco) is of concern, as this is being marketed and sold to children as a sweet.

What does oral cancer screening involve?

There are three main stages to oral cancer screening:

1 Raising awareness of oral cancer and the risk factors.
2 Encouraging patients to reduce their risk factors (for example, smoking cessation).
3 Regular visual and palpatory examinations of the oral soft tissues and lymph nodes.

Raising awareness of oral cancer and the risk factors and reducing their risk

It is helpful to use simple language. The term 'mouth cancer' is more readily understood by patients. Patient literature (for example, British Dental Health Federation (BDHF) or in-house practice leaflets) is a good way of starting to increase patient awareness and understanding of oral cancer and its associated lifestyle risk factors. Medical history sheets can include questions on alcohol and tobacco use. This will help elicit as much relevant detail as possible. However, this information should be reinforced on a one-to-one basis, particularly for those patients with one or more risk factors.

Cancer is a potentially emotive subject, and patients will react in many different ways, from absolute denial or indifference, to unnecessary overconcern.

You will help ease the patients' concerns if you are prepared for likely questions and reactions, and can answer them in a way that each patient will understand. Patients will often ask the nurse or receptionist questions that they feel unable to ask you, so it is helpful if your team is equally able to answer patient queries and to reinforce lifestyle advice about reducing risk factors.

Patients should be encouraged to give up smoking, with support from sources such as Quitline (0800 002200). The Health Education Authority has published a booklet, *Helping Smokers to Stop – a guide for the dental team*, which gives useful and practical information to help patients ultimately reduce their risk of developing oral cancer.

Medical histories and dental records

Record both positive and negative findings from medical and lifestyle histories and update changes at each examination.

Dental records can include a pictorial mouth map (available from the BDA), which clearly indicates that each anatomical area has been examined and palpated. Any suspicious (benign or pre-cancerous) lesions must be accurately marked and compared against previous and subsequent records. Intra-oral photographs are especially useful when monitoring these lesions, and also for recording stained areas if OraTest is used (*see* p. 110).

The clinical examination procedure

To be successful this must be followed for every patient, rather than just known risk groups.

Work out a systematic examination procedure that works for both you and your nurse and stick to it. Document all your findings both positive and negative.

Perform a visual inspection of the face and neck as you appraise the patient's general well-being, not forgetting ears and bald heads for sun damage. Patients prefer examination of the lymph nodes of the neck before your gloves are wet with saliva. A systematic approach to lymph-gland examination should be routine for every GDP.

Remove all dentures prior to the intra-oral examination

You may wish to review certain patients more frequently, but for most, an annual routine oral cancer screen will suffice.

However, remember that every time you see a patient in your surgery is an opportunity to review their soft tissues. Similarly, you should advise your hygienist to be vigilant for unexplained mucosal changes, especially in patients with known risk factors for oral cancer.

The BDA has two videos that may be useful to enhance and develop your clinical examination skills:

- *The Importance of Being Early: dentists' responsibilities in relation to pre-malignancy and malignancy of the oral mucosa.*
- *Oral Cancer: a case for screening.*

A fourth stage is available to dental practitioners: the adjunctive use of tolonium chloride (also called toluidine blue and marketed in the UK as OraTest). OraTest is a mouthrinse which is easy to use and stains abnormal cells blue; it can detect lesions before they are visible to the human eye. Prior to using this technique you must fully understand its use, be able to interpret your results, and remember that it is in no way a substitute for a full clinical examination. OraTest can be offered as an adjunct to this clinical examination, although a private fee will have to be charged as it is not available under the NHS.

What to do if you find a suspicious lesion

Understand the procedures yourself, as your uncertainty would add to the patient's concerns and may delay referral. Familiarise yourself with the protocols of your practice and local maxillofacial unit.

The referral must be arranged as soon as possible; if you suspect a cancer, your referral should be sent via your local maxillofacial unit's fast-track system. The patient will be seen on a consultant clinic within two weeks if this system is used. Find out the fax number and keep it handy.

For less-urgent conditions write as usual, giving all relevant information so that the patient can be given an appropriate appointment. On arrival at a new practice, you may wish to write to the consultant to introduce yourself and clarify these procedures.

People are obviously very concerned about the possibility of having cancer. It is very important to offer support and honest reassurance. Phrases such as 'I don't know what it is Mrs Smith, that's why I need you to see the specialist' are non-alarmist and truthful (only a microscope can tell exactly what the lesion is). Explain that the first visit will probably be a consultation; however, the biopsy procedure can be described to prepare the patient for their hospital visits.

Include in your referral letter:

- patient personal details
- relevant medical history
- relevant lifestyle factors
- brief details of counselling provided and perceived level of patient understanding
- brief dental history
- details of the suspicious area/lesion (colour, texture, size, position, mobility)
- whether any regional nodes are palpable
- copy of all available mouth maps and photographs
- mention use of tolonium chloride if applicable.

If the biopsy confirms cancer, it is important to maintain open communications with the patient and continue to offer support as may be required. Following treatment, the patient will invariably have changed dental needs such as prosthetic appliances, post-radiation xerostomia and reduced blood supply to the oral regions. You must be aware of their implications to future treatments and plans.

You, your practice and oral cancer screening

As with many health issues, it is the patient's responsibility to reduce their risk of oral cancer. However, as a primary healthcare provider, it is your responsibility to empower them with the information and the encouragement to adapt their lifestyles and reduce the risk factors which are associated with the development of oral cancer. It follows that you must always be vigilant for early signs of oral cancer in order to give your patients the best opportunity for effective treatment and cure.

You may wish to discuss introducing a practice-based oral cancer screening programme with the practice owner and other members of staff. Introducing a comprehensive oral cancer screening programme throughout the practice will provide your patients with a high-quality service, which they will value. This in turn will positively promote your practice within the local community. The practice should certainly consider raising the general awareness of oral cancer, the associated risk factors, the importance of early detection and of a regular clinical examination.

One effective way to do this is to support Mouth Cancer Awareness Week which is a professional and public awareness campaign organised each year by the British Dental Health Foundation (www.dentalhealth.org.uk).

Top tips

- Find out how to refer for specialist advice and keep the fax/ phone numbers to hand.
- Remember to look at the face and neck, to identify lesions and assess well-being.

- Learn how to examine a neck and do it routinely for every patient.
- Practice your soft-tissue examination, and use it on every patient.
- Update medical and lifestyle history at every examination.
- Remember that non-smokers and young people can get mouth cancer.

Conclusions

- All dentists have an ethical and professional duty to provide the best dental and oral care and treatment for all their patients.
- Oral cancer screening should become part of every routine examination appointment.
- Patients (and also the wider local community) should be made aware of the risk factors associated with the development of oral cancer.
- Ethnic groups should be made aware of the specific risks of using chewing tobacco.
- Early diagnosis is critical to reducing the morbidity and mortality rates of oral cancer.
- General dental practitioners should be aware of the changed dental needs of patients with oral cancer (treatment planning, post-treatment side-effects).

Further information

- BDA occasional paper, *Oral Cancer: guidelines for early detection*. Occasional Paper 5 (May 1998). British Dental Association, London.

- BDA occasional paper, *Opportunistic Oral Cancer Screening.* Occasional Paper 6 (2000). British Dental Association, London. *A management strategy for oral cancer screening in general dental practice.*
- For professional and patient information material and administrative guidelines call Zila Europe on Freephone 0800 028 23 33.

Section 7

8 Your practice

Introduction

In essence a dental practice is like any business in its management and financial aspects. While clinical aspects are obviously of paramount importance, lack of attention to the business side of the practice can have serious consequences for the practitioner who is not protected from the normal commercial considerations merely by the nature of his/her chosen profession.

Indeed the increasingly competitive nature of dentistry, with its restriction on national health funding and the pressures to attract more patients through the projection of a high-quality image, has meant that serious attention to running a sound financial business has become more important than ever.

It is hoped that this section of the manual will cover a number of key areas critical to a successful start in your own practice, or to selecting the right associateship.

Location

Selecting the right location is an extremely important factor in your first practice project as it will need to offer both good business potential and an environment in which you are happy to work, and perhaps live in.

The following is a list of some of the factors to be considered in selecting a favoured area:

- personal preference – rural, city, suburban
- dentist/patient ratio (local health authority can provide information)
- economic factors in the area
- population – static, declining, increasing, young, old?
- property values – future planned developments (local authority planning department).

Premises

Several different types of property may be available in the area, for example the opportunity to purchase freehold premises, or a leasehold arrangement might be possible. From a financial standpoint, combining the practice with your home can often be an attractive option in the early years, but could prove a burden in later years, as the Inland Revenue will look at the capital gains made by the business aspect of the premises. Currently you do not pay capital gains tax on any gain from your personal domicile.

Here are some of the factors to think about:

- cost both of freehold and leasehold
- professional valuations
- security of tenure if rented or leasehold
- availability of surgery space
- parking
- view or setting
- opportunities for expansion
- proximity of other services
- quality of environment

- local transport system
- but most importantly the patient list or potential.

The business plan

In order that you have a structure to refer to and a measure against which to judge performance, it is essential that a formal business plan – stating your present and future intention – be compiled. This will also be vital if you intend approaching sources from which to raise finance for your project. At this point you should retain the services of a good accounting firm, preferably one with experience of the dental profession. This will ensure that your business plan, including a first-year budget and cash-flow forecast, is correctly put together in a businesslike fashion.

This business plan should cover the following areas:

- personal requirements
- your objectives and goals
- why you have selected the particular area
- physical resources
- capital expenditure requirements
- first-year budget showing expected income/overheads
- first-year cash flow showing monthly movement of money
- anticipated future expansion potential.

You should use the business plan to 'sell' your business plan to your backers, be they banks, PCTs or finance companies.

The business plan should include your vision, where you want to be and what you want your business to be about. It should also incorporate your mission and what your business actually does.

Remember to look at personnel aspects, your staff, how you will train them and help them meet the goals and objectives of your business.

Finance

Your business plan will assist you in approaching lenders from whom you may wish to borrow funds to assist your plans. There is no shortage of banks, insurance companies and finance houses competing for this business; indeed some finance houses have specialised operations to cater specifically for dentists. It is important that you have the right loan, from the right lender, and here again your accountants should be able to provide impartial advice. The sources likely to provide finance are as follows:

- property – banks, insurance companies, building societies
- renovation/refurbishment costs – as above plus finance houses
- equipment – banks, finance houses
- working capital (overdraft) – banks.

Management

Even the best-planned operations often fail due to bad management and so in addition to paying close attention to clinical skills and requirements, it is imperative that every care is taken in how you manage your practice or, in other words, your business. You will have to review the following key areas:

- clinical management
- administration management
- financial management
- staff management.

In the dental world it is impossible to get away from having to market the practice. In fact it is imperative that a practice 'sells' itself, as no growth is likely without such action. Key areas of the marketing function are:

- planning and achieving growth
- motivation planning
- creating the dental care team within your practice
- image building
- postgraduate education
- patient communication/information within the practice

Think about the seven Ps.

- People – who you employ, who you treat.
- Place – where you provide your service, customer service.
- Product – what you provide.
- Physical evidence – the premises, the ambience, the staff, the 'brand'.
- Promotion – how you 'sell/promote' your services.
- Process – how you actually take a person from first contact to completion of treatment.
- Price – what it costs!

There are increasingly a number of courses aimed at giving dentists a broader range of business skills.

Bristol University run the BUOLD (Bristol University's Open Learning for Dentists) course which results in a recognisable postgraduate qualification, the DPDS (Diploma in Postgraduate Dental Studies). This is a modular course with each candidate required to complete three modules over five years. The modules consist of written homework assignments and an examination at the end. One of these modules is the Business Management Skills for Dentists which provides a thorough overview to MBA (Master of Business Administration) level of the skills needed for managing a dental practice.

More information can be obtained from:

BUOLD Co-ordinator
BUOLD Course Applications
Dental Postgraduate Department
The Chapter House
Lower Maudlin Street
Bristol BS1 2LY

Practice finance

The fundamental requirement to equip a practice is at the heart of every dentist's professional life. Given the competitive business world that dentists now find themselves in, along with enhanced patient expectations and the rapid pace of technological advance in equipment, it can be seen that the financial requirements needed to operate a modern dental practice can be somewhat daunting.

Selecting the right source of funding that is appropriate for each element of a particular surgery project is often critical to the long-term financial health of a practice. If arranging finance for professional people were as simple as providing rates and repayment periods it would be a very straightforward business indeed, but simple it simply is not. Everyone's needs and circumstances are different and, unless they are understood fully, financial advice can be given that is horrifyingly wide of the mark. So selecting the right type of finance and the right organisation to provide it is critical.

Banks

The main area served by the clearing banks in addition to providing day-to-day cash and cheque paying facilities is in the area of loans for practice purchase. These are usually on a secured basis and endowments and pension plans are often used to provide very tax-efficient repayment facilities. The dentist's bank may also provide loans for surgery improvements and working capital usually in the form of overdrafts, which are necessary for the day-to-day working of the practice. The bank will also be involved with personal banking requirements outside the practice area.

However, in order to prevent overloading bank facilities, many dentists avail themselves of more specialised forms of finance when it comes to funding their equipment and other major practice assets, i.e. computers, furnishings, business systems, etc. This type of finance is usually accessed from finance companies and usually comes in the form of either leasing or hire purchase and is unsecured and relatively short term in line with the effective useful life of the equipment.

Finance houses

Hire purchase

This entails financing the cost of equipment over a set period of time and paying for it in fixed monthly instalments.

Hire purchase has always been popular because it gives ultimate ownership. Tax relief is available in the form of writing down allowances, currently at 25% per annum, on a reducing balance basis. The practical effect of this is to spread tax relief over a somewhat lengthy period of time, often over ten years, which is usually much longer than the term of the loan and probably longer than the optimum life of the equipment.

Leasing

Leasing allows the use of equipment over a set time period at fixed monthly rentals but without ultimately owning the asset.

Leasing currently offers the dentist greater tax efficiency as tax relief is given by allowing the total annual rental payment as a practice expense at the dentist's highest tax rate. The total amount of tax relief is thus obtainable within the term of the lease, usually three, four or five years giving the dentist the full benefit of that relief much sooner than the hire purchase or indeed any other method of purchase such as a bank loan.

A much-used criticism of leasing is that the lessee never owns the equipment. This is true and would be a valid point were the equipment in question to be an appreciating asset where ownership would obviously be an advantage. However, with most dental equipment the opposite is the case and it could be argued that ownership merely prolongs the use of outdated, inefficient and non-cost-effective equipment.

Finance companies

A number of specialised finance companies operate within the dental market offering many options to suit practitioners' requirements. Special payment profiles to assist new growing practices or to overcome particular tax problems can be constructed, and built-in insurance protection is also available with some leasing and hire purchase plans on offer.

In general, dentists are still regarded by financial institutions as a below-average risk, but in today's fast-moving business world automatic approval of one's plans cannot be taken for granted. Institutions will look for a dentist beginning a new surgery project to demonstrate competence and a business-like attitude in order to justify borrowings which in many cases can amount to tens of thousands of pounds. The provision of a comprehensive and detailed business plan will usually be a prerequisite for any significant borrowing application and the construction of this is detailed elsewhere in this manual.

The role of the accountant

Having qualified as a dentist, you are a professional person who now has to learn how to operate in a commercial and business world where you will normally look to become an associate, partner or sole principal running a business to make a profit.

Other taxation matters

- Have you declared all sources of your income, including cash fees, sale of dental accessories, waste materials etc?
- How do national insurance contributions (NIC), value-added tax, capital gains tax or inheritance tax affect you, your family and your business?
- How do you obtain tax relief on capital expenditure, equipment, property and computers?
- Would leasing of equipment be more beneficial rather than outright purchase?
- Are you applying the PAYE (pay as you earn)/NIC rules correctly to your staff and you?

Hence you will need to seek advice from an accountant to help you make certain business decisions, explain the complexities of the taxation system and how to manage your business affairs. It is vital that you use an accountant that is specialised in the dental profession and is aware of the latest changes and financial procedures that exist in the profession.

In this section, we will cover a number of important considerations to help ensure that you obtain a strong financial team of advisors for your future career.

The vocational dental practitioner

As a vocational dental practitioner (VDP), there is no need for you to employ an accountant, but as your VDP year draws to an end, it is wise to consider finding one who will assist you in preparing associate agreements and will offer early advice on accounts and business records. Please remember it is important to keep records of:

- professional subscriptions
- car expenses and mileage
- telephone accounts
- expenses solely connected with work
- full business income and fees from all sources
- courses
- NHS superannuation.

This will reduce the accountant's work and thus his or her charges. A first year accountant's bill for an associate should be about £400, but could be much higher, if proper records are not maintained.

Full accounting records for your business must be maintained. The Inland Revenue imposes a maximum fine of £3000 if you fail to do so.

When you become an associate, it is important to remember that you are not taxed at source, but will be liable to pay tax some time after the year end. You should save approximately 25% of your earnings for this, but your accountant can advise.

Class 2 national insurance has to be paid monthly – preferably by a direct debit monthly arrangement – but an additional amount will be payable based on profits (Class 4) chargeable at the end of the tax year, or a penalty can result with no right of appeal if time limits are not met.

How income tax affects you

This is the difference between being an employee – subject to Schedule E and automatic tax and NIC deduction – and being self-employed – subject to Schedule D and accounting for your own taxes and NIC.

You will need an accountant to advise on:

- the dates your taxes become payable
- how your taxes are calculated
- what expenses are allowable
- what income is taxable
- the basis of assessing your income
- what records should be maintained for both income and outgoings

Under the present tax system you will have to 'self-assess' your tax and national insurance liabilities for each complete tax year.

How national insurance affects you

- This is effectively an additional form of taxation of which there are four types: Class 1, Class 2, Class 3 and Class 4.
- It is quite possible for you to be liable to Classes 1, 2 and 4 at the same time and careful consideration to exceptions or deferment must be given.
- Do you know how to make the appropriate election? Your accountant should.
- It is ultimately your responsibility to organise your tax and NIC affairs and make your payments when due. There are interest and penalty charges if you get it wrong, with no right of appeal.

Practice management

Efficient and effective management in the following key areas can enhance your profits:

- efficient book-keeping systems
- computer application
- credit control for patient charges and private patient fees
- control of expenditure
- maximising income
- budgeting and cash-flow forecasts
- employment of a good practice manager/financial secretary
- financial capital outlay – comparison of different methods
- terms for dental associates
- do you require locum or other assistance?

Your accountant can provide crucial advice in all these areas and should provide an annual practice performance review as part of their normal service.

Associate and partnership agreements and changes

When dealing with these agreements you should consider, with your accountant, the following:

1 Contents – particularly admission and retirement, methods of valuation, capital to be introduced or withdrawn, percentage profit shares, and the basis on which they are computed, and how disputes are resolved.
2 Which expenses are to be borne solely from your fees earned?
3 Which expenses are to be pooled?

4   Profit and capital shares and future increases.
5   Compliance with self-assessment taxation systems.

Introduction to personal and practice insurance and investment

As a dental surgeon you will in most cases become the operator, owner or part-owner of a business. Other sections of the guide confirm the need for specialist accountancy and finance (equipment purchase) advice; likewise, the need for timely and accurate advice in relation to insurance and investment both in relation to your personal and practice requirements will be absolutely vital.

You have embarked on a career that will bring many rewards, not least of them financial. It is important to remember however that you are uniquely dependent on good health and fitness to carry out your chosen profession. Accident, sickness or major illness can and does strike, any of which could render you unable to work on a short-, medium- or long-term basis. How will bills be paid? How will any family be supported? How will practice expenses be catered for? And, last but not least, how will I fund my eventual retirement without or on a reduced income? These are all questions that you should ask yourself throughout your career, but especially during the early years when adequate cover can be purchased most cheaply with the least amount of fuss.

Who can advise me?

At one time the insurance industry sold a few very similar insurance products mostly through individual company sales forces. Originally they could and did advise on other company products. With the advent of the Financial Services Act 1986 all this changed in that a company representative was then only allowed to discuss the products of his or her own company. From then on to obtain market-wide advice you had to employ the services of an IFA (independent financial advisor).

The IFA sector has grown from a tiny proportion of market share to approaching 50% since the Financial Services Act (FSA) 1986. Financial products have become more and more complex requiring specific advice over a wide range of needs and topics. It has been increasingly recognised by the industry and a growing number of professionals that it is now only possible to obtain the best advice from an IFA specialising in the individual's own profession. In short you need an independent advisor who has many dentists already as clients and therefore should be aware of and able to advise you on all the specialist products and investments that are most suitable for dentists. You will often be placed under pressure from banks, building societies and estate agents to purchase their products. Always have such proposals checked by an independent advisor to ensure they are adequate and/or suitable to your profession. Make sure you are aware who your advisor represents and how he or she is being paid.

In what areas do I need advice now?

Initially you should ensure that you have adequate protection insurance in place. Retirement and savings plans can be considered when affordable. In any event you should always remember that delay will inevitably increase the cost of most insurance and investment products, especially retirement plans. You and your financial advisor should always ensure that any plans you take up are affordable and in the correct order of priority. Normally replacement income (personal health insurance), critical illness cover and life cover should be your first considerations subject to your individual needs. Make sure the policy you take out has the right amount of cover, maximum events (risks) covered and no exclusions relative to dentists.

Which companies should I use?

As previously discussed, be guided by an experienced IFA; however, be sure to consider the advantages of using companies like the Dentists' Provident Society and Dentists & General. Any advisor you take on should be able and willing to advise on these companies. Many are not.

The Dentists' Provident Society (DPS) was founded in 1908 by dentists for dentists and membership is restricted to those on the dentists' register or those on the medical register with dental qualifications. They are a registered 'friendly society' and offer excellent day one cover plus a tax-free lump sum on retirement based on the number of basic (investment) shares held. Subscriptions are, unusually, the same for both sexes (females often pay more) and there is no exclusion for HIV (human immunodeficiency virus) or AIDS-related conditions. Special terms are available for vocational trainees. Currently payments in claim reduce to 50% at 26 weeks and 30% at 52 weeks; however, they are hoping to offer non-reducing benefits shortly.

Dentists & General offer very similar benefits in a similar format to those of DPS with the addition of a deferred benefit that can be useful in making up the shortfall when the DPS scheme reduced at 26 and 52 weeks respectively. Historically their with-profit returns, although good, have not surpassed those of DPS. They are not exclusive to dental surgeons.

Essential steps on qualification

1   Registration with General Dental Council.
2   Enrol as a member of a defence union or society.
3   Consider carefully basic income protection for VDPs as appropriate (provides income protection beyond guaranteed four weeks for VDPs).
4   Joining the British Dental Association and the Faculty of General Dental Practitioners is highly recommended.

Essential steps on becoming an associate

1   Obtain the services of a dental-specific accountant.
2   Obtain the services of a dental-specific finance broker for car or equipment purchase.
3   Obtain the services of a dental-specific IFA.
4   Consider best options for income protection, critical illness and disability cover. Life cover, retirement and savings plans could be considered where appropriate and affordable.
5   Arrange practice expenses cover if you are liable for any proportion of them.

Essential steps on practice purchase or becoming a partner

1   Review the performance of all your advisors. Change them if you do not believe they can provide adequate support in the execution of your plans.
2   Take out revenue investigation insurance cover.

3   Consider all finance options – secured, unsecured, etc.

4   Take out locum or practice expenses cover.

5   Ensure you have a correctly worded legal partnership agreement if taking on a partner.

6   If in partnership take out adequate partnership assurance with ideally a critical illness element.

7   Re-evaluate and adjust where necessary all your protection arrangements and financial planning.

8   Pay special attention to retirement planning if your income is derived mostly from private practice or likely to become so.

Look after your dental rep

Many dentists do not make any time to see dental representatives when they call at a practice. They may be someone from an established or a new dental company but, whichever, there are so many benefits to inviting a dental rep into your practice. Of course, the dental rep is likely to be on a mission to sell you new materials, equipment or services. To have the opportunity to keep abreast of changes in our profession there is no harm in offering a cup of coffee, a little hospitality and about 20 minutes of your time. It is your choice as to what to do after weighing up the benefits about the new product or service.

Additionally, you can find that dental reps are a great source of knowledge about the dental community and can be extremely helpful regarding staff recruitment (someone looking for a new job), how to dispose of old equipment, such as taking it to the excellent dental charity, Dentaid (supporting dentistry in the third world – www.dentaid.org.com).

Although you may not buy from a dental rep when they visit, you are challenging your scientific understanding and general practice experiences in assessing their wares. You could even record these visits as non verifiable continuing professional development (CPD). When you take on a large project such as building or equipping a dental practice then you are likely to gain advice regarding design and project management.

To summarise, by looking after your dental rep you can:

- learn about new materials and dental trends
- save time and expense as merchandise is brought to you
- gain insight into your local dental community
- open doors for new staff or even new premises
- challenge and keep scientific knowledge up to date
- offer advice for disposal of equipment
- record the visits as a source of potential CPD
- design resource and project management advice for large projects.

Dental surgery design

There are several major issues relating to dental surgery design. It is important to achieve the optimum working environment for the dental team and the most relaxed situation for the patient ensuring that a clinical procedure is as comfortable as possible for everyone involved. This, for the most part, means placing the important items within easy reach, allowing the procedure to be carried out with the least amount of disruption and within the minimum time.

Many situations offer compromise due to room constraints, supply of services, existing equipment and budget or specialist requirements. However, if you start with the ideal in mind and work to this as closely as possible, it must be better than leaving it to chance. How would you arrive at the ideal? In most instances the clinician will have a good idea of what to look for. There are many advantages to calling in the experts. There are people who design dental surgeries every day and therefore have the expertise to advise and guide you toward a more ergonomic layout, while still accommodating any other constraints. Within the British Dental Trade Association (www.bdta.org.uk) there is a wealth of knowledge and experience to be found.

Other considerations may be aesthetics, patient flow, and flexibility for multiple users, natural and artificial lighting and future issues relating to technology and regulations. Unfortunately most projects start with budget as the highest priority, when function, reliability and longevity should be of greater importance.

Where you start is dependent upon whether you are looking to totally refurbish, or to simply upgrade. With total refurbishment the optimum would be a blank room which allows the location of services (plumbing and electrical) anywhere within. You would first choose a cabinetry design based upon the proposed use. Is the surgery required to work for both left- and right-handed operators? This is one of the first and most topical issues of the day. Over 15% of the current population of dental schools are left-handed. Several dental equipment manufacturers have taken this into account and offer ambidextrous packages.

It is a good idea to sketch out the surgery design on the floor of the room to be equipped and simulate inviting a patient into the dental chair and working with your nurse within this 'new space'. Architects, designers and dentists can become distracted by artistry and innovation and can miss obvious important and practical issues. Being involved with designing a dental surgery can be a very rewarding and insightful time regarding the way you work and they way you would like to work.

Section 8

Further information

Directory of major dental supply companies

Key to company codes

A General supplies, materials, instruments, etc.

B Equipment manufacturers – dental chairs, etc.

C Dental stationery – letterheads, forms, stickers, etc.

D Dental pharmaceuticals, dentifrices, toothbrushes, etc.

E Surgery furniture.

F Finance, leasing.

G Oral cancer detection.

H Periodontal therapy products.

I Implantology.

J Dental bodies – corporate.

3M ESPE Dental Products
Unit 10
Beazer Court
Belton Road West
Loughborough
Leicestershire LE11 5TR

Tel: 01509 613361

www.3mespe.com

A

Admor Ltd
Kings Close
Yapton
West Sussex BN18 0EX
Tel: 01243 553078
www.admor.co.uk
C

British Dental Trade Association
Mineral Lane
Chesham
Bucks HP5 1NL
Tel: 01494 782873
Fax: 01494 786659
Email: admin@bdta.org.uk
www.bdta.org.uk
A to K

Campbell Montague International Limited (CMI)
Number 9 Berkeley Street
London W1J 8DW
Tel: 020 7297 4500
Fax: 020 7495 2950
www.cmi.uk.com
F

Castellini Ltd
5 Hawkley Brook Estate
Worthington Way
Wigan WN3 6XE
Tel: 01942 237 959

Fax: 01942 245 809
Email: Castellini@aol.com
www.castellini.com
B

Clark Dental
6 Victory Close
Fulmar Way
Wickford Business Park
Essex SS11 8YW
Tel: 01268 733146
B

Claudius Ash/J & S Davis
Summit House
Summit Road
Cranborne Industrial Estate
Potters Bar
Herts EN6 3EE
Tel: 01707 646330
A

Colgate Oral Pharmaceuticals
Guildford Business Park
Middleton Road
Guildford
Surrey GU2 8SZ
Tel: 01483 302222
www.colgate.co.uk
D

Denplan Ltd
Denplan Court
Victoria Road
Winchester

Hampshire SO23 7RG
Tel: 01962 828 000
www.denplan.co.uk
J

The Dental Directory
Billericay Dental Supply Co. Ltd
6 Perry Way
Witham
Essex CM8 3SX
Tel: 01376 500222
www.dental-directory.co.uk
A

DENTSPLY Ltd
Hamm Moor Lane
Addlestone
Weybridge
Surrey KT15 2SE
Tel: 01932 853422
www.dentsply.co.uk
A

Dexcel Dental
1 Cottesbrooke Park
Heartlands Business Park
Daventry
Northants NN11 5YL
Tel: 01327 312266
www.dexcelpharma.com
H

FORESTADENT UK
21 Carters Lane
Kiln Farm

Milton Keynes
Buckinghamshire MK11 3HL
Tel: 01908 568 922
www.forestadent.co.uk
A

Johnson & Johnson Ltd
Dental Care Division
Foundation Park
Roxborough Way
Maidenhead
Berkshire SL6 3UG
Tel: 01628 822222
A

KaVo Dental Ltd
Raans Road
Amersham
Bucks HP6 6JL
Tel: 01494 733000
www.kavo.com
B

Kent Express Ltd
Medcare House
Centurion Close
Gillingham Business Park
Gillingham
Kent ME8 0BR
Tel: 01634 878787
www.kentexpress.co.uk
A

Minerva Dental Ltd
Unit 3, Liberty Industrial Park

South Liberty Lane
Bristol BS3 2SU
Tel: 0117 963 2874
Fax: 0117 963 7984
www.minervadental.co.uk
A

Nobel Biocare
Nobel House
The Grand Union Office Park
Packet Boat Lane
Uxbridge
Middlesex UB8 2GH
Tel: 01895 430650
www.nobelbiocare.com
I

Oasis Dental Care
69–75 Thorpe Road
Norwich NR1 1UA
Tel: 08000 324466
www.oasisdentalcare.com
J

Oral-B Laboratories
Gillette Corner
Great West Road
Isleworth TW7 5NP
Tel: 020 8847 7817
D

Takara Belmont (UK) Ltd
Belmont House
1 St Andrews Way
Bow
London E3 3PA

Tel: 020 7515 0333
www.takara.co.uk
B

SS White Ltd
9 Madleaze Estate
Bristol Road
Gloucester GL1 5SG
Tel: 01452 307171
www.sswhite.com
A

Wright Health Group Ltd
Dunsinane Avenue
Kingsway West
Dundee DD2 3QD
Tel: 01382 833866
A, B, D, E

Zila Inc.
5227 North 7th Street
Phoenix, AZ 85014–2800
Tel: 001 602 266 6700
www.zila.com
G

Useful addresses

Association of Dental Anaesthetists of Great Britain and Ireland
21 Portland Place
London W1B 1PY
Tel: 020 7631 1650
www.aagbi.org

BDA – British Dental Association
64 Wimpole Street
London W1M 8AL
Tel: 020 7935 0875
www.bda.org

BDDG – British Doctors and Dentists Group (alcohol related help group)
3 St Andrew's Place
Regent's Park
London NW1 4LB
Tel: 020 7487 4445
Fax: 020 7935 4479
Email: mca@medicouncilalcol.demon.co.uk
www.medicouncilalcol.demon.co.uk

BDHF – British Dental Health Foundation
Smile House
2 East Union Street
Rugby
Warwickshire CV22 6AJ
Tel: 0870 770 4000
www.dentalhealth.org.uk

BDTA –British Dental Trade Association
Mineral Lane
Chesham
Bucks HP5 1NL
Tel: 01494 782873
www.bdta.org.uk

BFS – British Fluoridation Society
Ward 4
Booth Hall Children's Hospital
Charlestown Road

Manchester M9 7AA
Tel/Fax: 0161 220 5223
Email: bfs@bfsweb.org
www.bfsweb.org/

BMA – British Medical Association
BMA House
Tavistock Square
London WC1H 9JP
Tel: 020 7387 4499
Fax: 020 7383 6400
www.bma.org.uk

D&G – The Dentists' and General Mutual Benefit Society
St James Court
20 Calthorpe Road
Edgbaston
Birmingham B15 1RP
Tel: 0121 452 1066
Fax: 0121 452 1077
www.dengen.co.uk

DPB – Dental Practice Board
Compton Place Road
Eastbourne
East Sussex BN20 8AD
Switchboard tel: 01323 417000
Helpdesk tel: 01323 433550
www.dpb.nhs.uk

DPL – Dental Protection Ltd
33 Cavendish Square
London W1M 0PS
Tel: 020 7399 1400
www.mps.org.uk

DPS – Dentists' Provident Society
9 Gayfere Street
Westminster
London SW1P 3HN
Tel: 020 7222 2511
www.dps-ltd.co.uk

FGDP – Faculty of General Dental Practitioners (UK)
The Royal College of Surgeons of England
35–43 Lincoln's Inn Fields
London WC2A 3PN
Tel: 020 7405 3474
www.rcseng.ac.uk/fgdp

GDC – General Dental Council
37 Wimpole Street
London W1M 8DQ
Tel: 020 7887 3800
www.gdc-uk.org

GDPA – General Dental Practitioners' Association
Dental Practitioners' Association
61 Harley Street
London W1G 8QU
Tel: 020 7636 1072
www.uk-dentistry.org/

Health Protection Agency
(merged with National Radiological Protection Board 1 April
2005)
Centre for Radiation, Chemical and Environmental Hazards
Chilton
Didcot
Oxon OX11 0RQ
Tel: 01235 831600
Email: rpd@hpa-rp.org.uk (Radiation Protection Division)
www.hpa.org.uk

MDDUS – Medical and Dental Defence Union of Scotland
Mackintosh House
120 Blythswood Street
Glasgow G2 4EA
Tel: 0141 221 5858
Fax 0141 354 1015
www.mddus.com

MDU – Medical Defence Union
MDU Services Limited
230 Blackfriars Road
London SE1 8PJ
Tel: 020 7202 1500
www.the-mdu.com

MIA – Medical Insurance Agency
The Bailey
PO Box 101
Skipton
North Yorkshire BD23 1XT
Tel: 0800 032 1896
www.mia.co.uk

MSS – Medical Sickness Society
Colmore Circus
Birmingham B4 6AR
Tel: 0800 197 0310
www.medical-sickness.co.uk

HA (local) health authority

....

....

....

....

BDA rep (local)

....

....

....

....

British Dental Association publications

The following advisory publications are available free of charge
to members of the British Dental Association. Non-members
may purchase the full set of advice sheets.

A   Practice management:
   A1   Planning Permission
   A2   Buying and Selling a Practice
   A3   Health & Safety Law for Dental Practice
   A4   Changing the (NHS/Private) Balance of Your Practice
   A6   Promoting Your Practice
   A7   Associateship Agreements
   A8   Employing an Assistant in General Practice
   A10 Partnership Agreements

A11 Radiation in Dentistry

A12 Infection Control in Dentistry

A13 Locumships in General Dental Practice

A14 Dentists' Maternity Arrangements and Pay

A15 Computers in General Practice

A16 Quality Management Using ISO 9002

A17 Practice Management Checklist

A18 Setting up in Practice

A19 Working with Dental Laboratories

B Ethical and legal:
   B1 Ethics in Dentistry

   B2 Data Protection

   B3 Giving Evidence

   B4 What to Do When a Practitioner Dies

   B5 Discipline Committee Arrangements

   B7 Practice Inspections

   B8 Did You Know? . . . Essential Legislation for General
        Practitioners

   B9 Prescribing in General Dental Practice

   B10 Handling Complaints

C Financial:
   C1 Sickness and Accident Insurance

   C2 Collecting Money from Patients

   C3 Business Plans

   C4 A Guide to Private Dental Schemes

   C5 Introduction to Taxation

   C6 Finance Management in General Dental Practice

   C7 Superannuation for NHS General Dental Practitioners

   C8 Fee Setting in Private Dental Practice

   C9 In-Practice Capitation Schemes

D Employing staff:
    D1 Contracts of Employment
    D2 Conditions of Employment for Dental Nurses
    D3 The Employment of Dental Hygienists
    D4 Conditions of Employment for Dental Technicians
    D5 Advice on the Direction of Dental Therapists
    D6 Pay for Dental Nurses in General Practice
    D7 Pay for Dental Hygienists in General Practice
    D8 Pay for Dental Technicians
    D9 Employees' Maternity Arrangements and Pay
    D10 Redundancy
    D11 Dismissal
    D12 Staff Recruitment
    D13 Discrimination in Employment
    D14 Violence at Work
    D15 Self-employed Hygienists

E Miscellaneous:
    E1 Working Abroad
    E3 Vocational Training in GDP
    E4 Guidance Notes for Part-time Teachers
    E5 Personal Dental Service
    E6 Developing Community Dental Services
    E7 A Guide to GDS Regulations
    E8 Working Abroad

S Students:
    S1 Help with Overseas Electives
    S2 Successful Interviews
    S3 Getting an Interview
    S4 Which Way Now – A Guide to Careers in Dentistry
    S5 Student Finances

Occasional papers

- *Oral Cancer – a guide to early detection.*
- *Oral Cancer – a management strategy for oral cancer screening in general dental practice.*

Information sheets

The BDA have a variety of information sheets from lists of accountants and solicitors, to notes on vocational training, peer review, private dental care plans and how to make a claim through the small claims court. If they haven't the information you need, they will try to compile it for you.

Other services

- Leaflets are also available on using the BDA member logo, on the BDA loan and on insurance and financial services through the BMA Services Limited. Three pads of 100 medical history sheets can be purchased.
- *At Your Service* – a directory of BDA services and whom to contact.

Should any topic of interest to you not be included in the BDA advice sheet list, or should any sheets be under revision or in preparation, telephone or write to the Membership Services Department, who will be pleased to advise you individually.

Your details

Name

Address

Phone number

Email

GDC registration number

Date of registration

Defence society

Defence society membership number

Defence society telephone number

NHS contract (performer) number

Primary Care Trust telephone number

BDA telephone number and email

BDA membership number

Other important telephone/email and website contacts

Index